A POSITIVE ENVIRONMENT?

PHYSICAL AND SOCIAL INFLUENCES ON PEOPLE WITH SENILE DEMENTIA IN RESIDENTIAL CARE

This book is dedicated to Cliff, Katie and Jo

A Positive Environment?

Physical and Social Influences on People with Senile Dementia in Residential Care

ANN NETTEN

PSSRU
UNIVERSITY OF KENT
AT CANTERBURY

Routledge
Taylor & Francis Group
LONDON AND NEW YORK

First published 1993 by Ashgate Publishing

Reissued 2018 by Routledge
2 Park Square, Milton Park, Abingdon, Oxon OX14 4RN
711 Third Avenue, New York, NY 10017, USA

Routledge is an imprint of the Taylor & Francis Group, an informa business

A Library of Congress record exists under LC control number: 92044396

Typeset at the PSSRU, University of Kent at Canterbury

ISBN 13: 978-1-138-60840-5 (hbk)
ISBN 13: 978-0-429-46341-9 (ebk)

Contents

Preface

My thanks are due to many people without whose advice, practical assistance and support this book would not have been possible. During the study Ann Clewer has provided invaluable support and advice, particularly of a statistical nature, and David Challis has been an excellent source of advice, obscure references and brainstorming sessions, especially at the start of the study. My thanks are also due to Bob Woods, who undertook the thankless task of external examiner, and Bleddyn Davies, whose support and encouragement have enabled the book to be completed.

If it had not been for the support of the Dora Harvey Memorial Trust the study would never have been initiated. The grant from this trust enabled me to undertake the doctoral programme: the fortuitous arrival of my application and this grant on the same desk on the same day will never cease to amaze me. Financial support was also received at a time of crisis from the Alzheimer's Disease Society. The cost of printing the instrumentation for the study exceeded the money available by (what seemed at the time) a huge sum. I shall always be grateful to the Society for their positive and speedy response to a request for help.

The data collection was the result of a lot of work from many people who were astoundingly co-operative in the face of what must have seemed like constant misrepresentation about the amount of time and effort required. In particular, the staff of the fifteen homes involved in the study (two pilot homes and thirteen in the main study) put in an enormous amount of time, effort and enthusiasm. The managerial staff in the social services departments were also unfailingly co-operative and helpful. My thanks are also due to the two social service managers who were prepared to give up their time for interview at the pilot stage.

Before I had access to a word processor, or any of the other benefits associated with being an employee of the PSSRU, several people provided secretarial help: Su Bellingham typed the questionnaires, Sandy Meggs typed letters and early versions of the literature review and pilot study, and Lucy Holley was a tremendous help in transferring the data on to the computer. Latterly, Anita Whitley has contributed with so many varied tasks (such as typing impossible tables, chasing references, photocopying and proof-reading) that I dare not try to identify them all for fear of omitting some. Jane Dennett has worked her customary miracle in converting the text into camera-ready copy and subediting.

I am grateful to Alan Sivell, who produced the diagrams for Chapter 5, and to Nick Brawn for photographing these, providing all the other diagrams and proof-reading. Figures 5.1 to 5.5 and Tables 5.1 to 5.3 first appeared in

Ann Netten, 'The effect of design of residential homes in creating dependency among confused elderly residents: a study of elderly demented residents and their ability to find their way around homes for the elderly' in the ***International Journal of Geriatric Psychiatry***, 1989, volume 4, pages 143-153 and are reprinted by kind permission of John Wiley & Sons Ltd. Moreover, Professor Rudolf Moos was most kind in giving permission to reproduce a table from the SCES manual.

Richard von Abendorff has been a great help in playing devil's advocate when discussing concepts and ideas. In the final tortuous stages of writing, rewriting and editing, Ann Clewer, David Challis, Cliff Netten, Helen Charnley and Jeni Beecham have been an enormous help in commenting on draft chapters. They have helped identify logical omissions, incomprehensible English and the more glaring grammatical errors. Justin Keen, Robin Lawson, Charlotte Salter and Justine Schneider have been most helpful in reading through later versions for sense and nonsense, and providing valuable comments on the contents.

The study would have been impossible to undertake in the absence of an effective, supportive, 'informal' network. I shall not try to list all the people who have helped in times of crisis, for fear of leaving someone out. However, I shall never forget the 'dry run' of the upgrading seminar with 'mathematical consultant' Mary McHale, 'media consultant' Phil McHale and 'bored onlooker' Cliff Netten. Lindsay Franklin, Mary McHale and Sherry Wilkin were a tremendous help in the early stages of child care arrangements. Gail Bayliff has been a reliable, flexible and uncritical 'mother's help' and friend. Only another working mother can truly appreciate the importance of that contribution. Last, but by no means least, Cliff, Katie and Jo have had to put up with a lot. Katie and Jo have been patient and understanding beyond their years and if it hadn't been for Cliff's contribution we would probably all be suffering from malnutrition.

Ann Netten
July 1992

1 Issues in the residential care of people with senile dementia

Like the prevalence of the disease itself, interest in residential care of people with senile dementia is bound to grow. While the option of domiciliary care may be achievable for increasingly high levels of disability, for other groups of elderly and disabled people there is a limit to the endurance of relatives and friends of people with dementia. Their demands are such that support provided by community-based social services is necessarily limited, and institutional care of some form frequently becomes the only viable option. It is important, both for those in receipt of care and for those who can no longer cope with the burden of care, that these institutions should provide the most beneficial environment possible.

The Wagner review of residential care took as a point of principle that:

> Living in a residential establishment should be a positive experience ensuring a better quality of life than the resident could enjoy in any other setting (Wagner, 1988, p.114).

But is it possible to determine if residents with senile dementia are having a positive experience? Is it possible to identify that they are enjoying a better quality of life than they could otherwise? Before such questions can be addressed there needs to be an understanding of the impact of different 'settings' or environments on elderly people with senile dementia. In particular there needs to be an understanding of the effect of the physical and social environment of the homes on the well-being of the 'confused' residents.

The focus of the investigation reported here is local authority residential care which caters for people of similar levels of disability to those cared for in both residential and nursing homes provided by the independent sector (Darton and Wright, 1989). The term 'residential care' is used throughout, but the discussion applies equally to nursing home accommodation. While the primary concern here is people with senile dementia, the problem to be addressed is the care of elderly people who have general orientation difficulties. Precise definitions are not of paramount importance. The category of resident with which this book is concerned is often termed 'confused'. Throughout, therefore, the terms 'confused', 'people with senile dementia', 'elderly mentally infirm people' and 'demented elderly people' are interchangeable.

Characteristics of dementia

Senile dementia can be described from a number of perspectives: technical medical descriptions of changes in the brain, psychological measures of types of memory loss, and so on. An operational definition of dementia has been given by the Royal College of Physicians Working Party on Organic Mental Impairment in the Elderly:

> Dementia is the global impairment of higher cortical functions including memory, the capacity to solve the problems of day-to-day living, the performance of learned perceptuo-motor skills, the correct use of social skills and control of emotional reactions in the absence of gross clouding of consciousness. The condition is often irreversible and progressive (Royal College of Physicians, 1981).

Dementia is defined, therefore, as symptoms and signs which may be the result of different pathological processes in the brain. Dementia can be described as pre-senile or senile depending on an arbitrary age limit (usually 65). Among senile dementias two conditions predominate:

- senile dementia of the Alzheimer type (SDAT), the commonest of all, is a primary degenerative disorder of the brain;
- multi-infarct dementia (MID) in which there is death of brain tissue (infarction) consequent upon a disorder of the cerebral circulation (haemorrhage, thrombosis or embolism).

An individual may suffer from either or both of these conditions. Unless there is a specific cause, such as a series of strokes, a firm diagnosis can be made only at autopsy. Diagnosis of dementia while the person is alive is a process of eliminating other possible causes such as the side-effects of drugs, alcoholism, urinary tract and chest infections, and other mental health problems (for example, depression).

Precise definitions and diagnoses of people suffering from senile dementia are desirable, but they are difficult to establish in the absence of clinical judgements. There are a number of diagnostic schemes such as the DSM III diagnostic criteria (American Psychiatric Association, 1980) which are used to determine the existence of dementia or Alzheimer's disease. There has been a lack of consistency in methods of assessment, which has led the Medical Research Council (1987) to recommend a set of minimum data to be collected in studies funded by the Council to aid comparison between research studies.

The concern here is primarily functional: to describe the observed changes in the individual. Gray and Isaacs (1979) describe the manifestation of brain failure as the individual displaying:

- a tendency to commit errors;
- a failure to perceive errors; and
- a failure to comprehend the consequences of errors.

The onset of dementia tends to be very gradual, with memory lapses often compensated for by writing notes or confabulation. To what extent compensatory mechanisms are related to the condition or to the personality of the individual has yet to be established (Woods and Britton, 1985). Referral usually occurs with the onset of more severe symptoms.

Holden and Woods point out that dementia is sometimes brought to the attention of professional care workers when an individual experiences a bereavement, change of house or other upheaval. Rather than being a causal factor:

Usually close examination reveals, for example, that the spouse who died was doing a great deal to compensate for the person's deficits that were developing before bereavement; the change of house removes a number of environmental props that were helping to sustain the person's failing functions, and so on (Holden and Woods, 1982, p.11).

Gray and Isaacs suggest seven symptoms which, although not comprehensive, most patients will show if observed long enough:

- lapses in personal hygiene, such as refusal to bathe;
- lapses in feeding and dressing, such as objectionable feeding habits;
- impairment of domestic skills, such as gas appliances turned on and not lit;
- lack of judgement and prudence, such as irresponsible expenditure of money;
- cognitive errors, such as failure to recognise close relatives;
- personality and interpersonal relations, such as groundless accusations; and
- miscellaneous offensive behaviour, such as verbal sexual advances.

These symptoms reflect the consequences of cognitive difficulties rather than the difficulties themselves, but provide a picture of the types of problem likely to be encountered by those caring for people with senile dementia.

By definition senile dementia is a progressive condition, and cognitive and behavioural difficulties are likely to increase with age. However, the pattern, both of behavioural difficulties and mental deterioration, varies from person to person. Personality changes sometimes occur, with some people becoming disinhibited, although others manage to carry on social conversations in spite of severe deterioration in mental abilities. Holden and Woods (1982) suggest that the rate of deterioration often seems slower when onset occurs in people in their 80s rather than in their 60s.

The difficulties in caring for people who display such behaviour that they become a danger to themselves and create embarrassment for others are often compounded by the demented person's failure to recognise the problem, as Sands and Suzuki point out:

Reifler et al. (1981) found that cognitively impaired persons living in the home saw themselves as suffering from no significant problems in activities of daily living, in personal health or in family relationships: professional persons and family care givers saw these same people as having problems in almost every area of life. For the person impaired this can lead to the feeling of being interfered with and manipulated; for the person giving care to feelings of being obstructed and unappreciated (Sands and Suzuki, 1983, p.21).

However, many people respond to the symptoms of senile dementia with anxiety and fear (Newroth and Newroth, 1980; Schwab et al., 1985). Holden and Woods (1982) also point out that not all patients lack this insight and that many are aware of deterioration and may complain of loss of memory. They state that it is not unusual for such people to show signs of anxiety and depression, perhaps in response to the repeated failures they experience.

Life expectancy is considerably reduced for people with dementia. Kay et al. (1970) found the mean expectation of life in patients over 65 reduced from 10.9 years to 2.3 years for women with senile dementia. For men, average life expectancy reduced from 8.7 years to 2.6 years. Similarly, 74 per cent of a sample of patients with senile dementia had died within 2.4 years compared with 26 per cent of a sample of mentally alert patients (Kay et al., 1970). Moreover, Roth (1955) found 60 per cent of demented patients had died within six months of admission to mental hospital compared to 11 per cent of those with affective psychosis. It is important, therefore, to distinguish carefully between organic and affective mental disorders whose expected outcomes are very different.

Although there is largely a consensus that the condition of senile dementia reduces life expectancy – although Christie (1985) has expressed reservations about the evidence – life expectancy among elderly people generally is rising. There has been some discussion in the literature regarding the supposed increase in the life expectancy of demented people in recent years, largely because of variations in results between individual studies. Thompson and Eastwood (1981) concluded there was no increase in life expectancy but their study suffered from the same problem as the others: inconsistency of definitions, especially in defining the onset of the condition. Frequently the date of admission is taken as the starting point, but admission policies tend to vary with internal and external pressures on services. Increased life expectancy among demented people may simply reflect improved nutrition generally and the use of antibiotics (Bergmann and Jacoby, 1982; Henderson, 1986). Immediate cause of death is often from another condition, such as bronchial pneumonia (Woods, 1989) so while there is no direct treatment for Alzheimer's disease itself, medical advances in other fields may affect the life expectancy of sufferers. Even if this is the case, however, it is not clear from the literature whether general increases in life expectancy will offset reductions due to dementia.

Incidence and prevalence

The problem of consistency of definitions also presents difficulties when discussing the incidence and prevalence of dementia. Mild, moderate and severe dementia are often distinguished but are rarely clearly defined other than in terms of instrumentation scores. Thus, 'mild' usually refers to people who are mildly confused or forgetful with no deterioration of personality or habits, 'severe' refers to considerable deterioration, and 'moderate' lies somewhere between the two.

Despite the problems of definition, a number of authors have drawn on individual studies of the prevalence of senile dementia to derive overall expected prevalence rates and future growth in this subpopulation. Preston (1986) used the data from seven studies and, adjusting for age differences, estimated that 6 per cent of those aged over 65 were likely to be moderately or severely demented. Ineichen (1987) also re-assessed a number of estimates of the incidence of dementia, including the Newcastle studies (Kay et al., 1964, 1970), examining assumptions and definitions. He concluded that 1 per cent of the 65-74 age group and 10 per cent of those over 75 suffer from dementia. Although these figures are lower than those of Kay et al. (1970) and Bergmann et al. (1978), they predict a larger rise in numbers given the expected population changes, so that between 1983 and 2001 there will be 17 per cent more people with senile dementia in England and Wales. In areas with high populations of elderly people, the increase will be much larger: during the same period the population of demented elderly people in the area served by Bath Health Authority is estimated to rise by 34 per cent. Other estimates put the increase in the numbers of people with senile dementia even higher. Using figures from Henwood and Wicks (1984), Sinclair (1988) predicted an increase of 52 per cent between 1971 and 2001 in Great Britain. This would mean an estimated 450,000 people had senile dementia in 1971 and this would rise to 684,000 by the year 2001. Similarly, using European-based age and gender prevalence rates estimated by Hofman et al. (1991), Schneider et al. (1992) used population projections to estimate that there were 540,000 people with dementia in England in 1991.

Such estimates, however, may be unduly pessimistic. A number of studies have identified a much lower prevalence than expected (Pattie et al., 1979; Clarke et al., 1986). O'Connor et al. (1989) report a rate of 5.3 per cent for moderate and severe dementia in a population aged 75 years and over. Using estimates by Jorm et al. (1987) these authors would have expected a prevalence of 11 per cent in this population. The authors suggest that the differences arise from using a more sensitive screening method (Cambridge Mental Disorders of the Elderly Examination, CAMDEX), rather than representing part of an overall cohort effect as has been proposed (Hagnell et al., 1981). Pattie (1988), in a discussion of similar results using Clifton Assessment Procedures for the Elderly (CAPE), suggests differences may be due to assumptions in earlier studies that 'mild' impairment would lead to severe dementia. Fries (1989) suggests that improved health and nutrition have resulted in the delay of onset of chronic illness so morbidity will be 'compressed' into a shorter period. He notes that there is insufficient evidence to say whether this is likely to be true of Alzheimer's disease. Henderson

(1986) has called for longitudinal studies using sensitive screening instruments to clarify prevalence rates.

It has been argued (Opit, 1988; Robertson, 1990) that much of the confusion about prevalence of mild dementia is to do with changing definitions. The separation of dementia from normal ageing processes is a social construct, culturally defined, and such definitions will shift with changes in the concerns of society. As mild confusional behaviour does not necessarily lead to severe senile dementia, the problem is not so much one of diagnosis as of boundary-setting.

Despite such debates there is little disagreement that the predominant risk factor of severe dementia is age. Kay et al. (1970) found that prevalence varied from 2.3 per cent in persons aged 60-69 to 22 per cent in those aged over 80. O'Connor et al. (1989) found 4.1 per cent of all grades of dementia in those aged 75 to 79, 11.3 per cent of those aged 80-84, 19.1 per cent of those aged 85 to 89, and 32.6 per cent in those aged 90 years or over. Even if the prevalence in the population as a whole is lower than thought, therefore, the ageing population ensures that severe senile dementia will continue to 'confront the world as a major challenge to public health' (Henderson, 1986, p.3).

The need for residential care

Independent living in the community and permanent hospitalisation represent the extreme ends of the spectrum in the 'continuum of care' (Knapp, 1984). In the policy world the emphasis is increasingly upon caring for people with physical and mental difficulties in the community. The aim is to shift care as far as possible towards the community end of the 'caring continuum' (Department of Health and Social Security, 1981; Griffiths, 1988).

A major consequence of the policy of shifting care of demented elderly people from institutions to the community will be an increased dependence upon carers and community-based services. Where carers are absent, community services may be able to provide adequate care for people who are physically dependent, but these services are unlikely to be able to fulfil the needs of otherwise unsupported elderly mentally infirm people. This is largely because of the constant level of monitoring which is required when caring for people whose judgement is poor and whose behaviour can be dangerous (Gray and Isaacs, 1979).

Even where carers are present, the stress of coping with senile dementia can have a profound effect (Sanford, 1975; Levin et al., 1983; Argyle et al., 1985). Gilleard (1982) found that over 50 per cent of a sample of 40 supporters of elderly mentally infirm people had significant psychological disturbances. Moreover, several studies using standard scales to measure morale or depression among carers of demented elderly people have found, that even when there is little evidence of psychiatric disturbance, morale is generally very low (Hirschfeld, 1978; Gilhooly, 1984).

Given the problems faced by carers of demented people, it is hardly surprising that the attitudes of carers have been found to be of fundamental importance in predicting admission to residential care, and carers are more likely to favour residential care if the elderly person is confused (Levin et al., 1989). There is also the issue of the future 'supply' of carers. Many carers are middle-aged women not in paid employment. Arber and Ginn (1990) analysed the OPCS informal carers survey and found that using the 'maximalist' definition the largest gender difference in caring occurs when people are in their late 40s. At this point, 25 per cent of women are carers compared with 15 per cent of men. An increase in the proportion of women in waged work together with an ageing population may reduce the proportion of elderly people who have carers willing and able to care for them at home (Parker, 1981).

There are limits, therefore, to the degree to which people with senile dementia can be cared for by the community (Argyle et al., 1985). In the representations made to an independent review of residential care (Wagner, 1988) the Alzheimer's Disease Society maintained that most people suffering from dementia would need residential care, be it long- or short-term, at some point in their lives. Moreover, the process of residential care is often seen as appropriate to the needs of people with senile dementia. West and his colleagues (1984) presented a series of vignettes to a large community sample in Scotland. In contrast to their attitude to elderly people with physical disability, two-thirds of the sample felt residential care was appropriate when the elderly person had a mental infirmity. It is not surprising, therefore, that in the mid-1980s while on average only about 5 per cent of elderly people were in some form of long-term institutional care (Kraan et al., 1991), Schneider et al. (1992), using the OPCS disability survey, estimated that 37 per cent of those with severe cognitive difficulties were cared for in residential or nursing facilities.

Sinclair (1988) concludes that the combination of carer strain and 'determined' community care policies resulting in closure of long-term geriatric and psychogeriatric wards is likely to result in an increasing proportion of confused people in local authority residential care. Although some observers have reservations about this prediction (Booth, 1983), the evidence to support this case is mounting.

Wilkin et al. (1978) found that between 1976 and 1977 there was an increase in residents with psychogeriatric problems in seven local authority homes, while three long-stay hospital wards experienced a reduction in such problems. The Personal Social Services Research Unit (PSSRU) at Kent also noted an increase in the proportion of residents with a confusional state: in 1981, 55 per cent of the residents of local authority homes had some confusional state compared with 44 per cent in the 1970 census (Darton,

1986b). By 1981, the behaviour of 22 per cent of the residents in the surveyed homes constituted a minor nuisance, and of 8 per cent a major nuisance. Mann et al. (1984) found that, in homes in Camden, two-thirds of residents had some form of confusional state and 38 per cent were depressed. Moreover, the residents could not be distinguished from long-term hospital patients in terms of dementia or dependency on staff. Similarly, Atkinson et al. (1986) reported the full range of mental confusion across private and local authority residential care, NHS nursing homes, and acute and geriatric wards in hospital. A survey of elderly people in receipt of health and social services in Waltham Forest found that a long-term policy of caring for elderly disabled people as far as possible in the community had resulted in local authority establishments 'providing primarily a dementia service' (Harrison et al., 1990, p.101). The authors found that only 13 per cent of 362 residents of local authority homes showed no evidence of dementia.

Just as the policy of community care puts residential care facilities under increasing pressure from a changing client population, the role of residential facilities is widening. For example, homes are being used more than ever for relief care: that is, short-term admissions to residential care in order to give relatives caring for them a break (Allen, 1983). Moreover, there is an increasing expectation of and trend towards homes acting as resource centres for the community (Barclay, 1982; Morton, 1991; Lawson, 1992). This confusion of status – whether residential care is about places or services – comes at a time when residential services, particularly in the statutory sector, are seen as a last resort, employing staff of low status and low morale (Wagner, 1988).

Residential care policy

Homes for elderly people were not originally intended to care for such a highly-dependent population (Health Advisory Service, 1982). The provision of modern residential care for elderly people is based on the Victorian workhouse. Under the Poor Law, in order to obtain support or benefit the claimant had to submit to a test under which homeless, rootless and penniless individuals were required to work in return for minimum assistance in an institution (Ministry of Health, 1955). The basis for this system did not change until after the second world war. Part III of the *National Assistance Act 1948* established a new basis for provision for old people no longer able to live independently in their own homes. This was envisaged in terms of 30-35 bedded homes, although a 1955 government review (Ministry of Health, 1955) suggested 60 beds might be more appropriate given the pressure on places. In an attempt to dispel the negative image of the workhouse, the emphasis was on a hotel model in which residents were encouraged to see themselves as guests. Even in the 1960s, however, Townsend (1962) found evidence of workhouse traditions. Since that time, the emphasis has been on representing that institution as the person's home. The gap between this aim and the reality has been the focus of various studies (for example, Evans et al., 1980; Willcocks et al., 1987).

Home Life: A Code of Practice for Residential Care (Centre for Policy on Ageing, 1984) was intended to provide a comprehensive set of requirements that should be met by establishments when providing residential care for a variety of client groups. This formed an integral part of the measures to regulate the establishment and conduct of private and voluntary care homes under the *Registered Homes Act 1984*. However, by December 1985 an independent review of residential care chaired by Lady Wagner was commissioned to:

> review the role of residential care and the range of services given in statutory, voluntary and private residential establishments within the personal social services in England and Wales; to consider, having regard to the practical constraints and other relevant developments, what changes, if any, are required to enable the residential sector to respond effectively to changing social needs; and to make recommendations accordingly (Wagner, 1988, p.1).

Both *Home Life* (Centre for Policy on Ageing, 1984) and *Residential Care: A Positive Choice* (Wagner, 1988) covered all types of residential care. Thus recommendations tended to be broad-based, and relatively few were directed towards the specific difficulties of people with senile dementia. In discussing the particular problems of dementia, Wagner stated that:

> The evidence of several inquiries and personal letters to the Committee underline the fact that where standards are not acceptable, the residents are caught in a downward spiral of confusion and disorientation (1988, p.112).

Fundamental aims of *Caring for People* (Cm 849, 1989) and the subsequent legislation (*National Health Service and Community Care Act 1990*) are to improve consumer choice and promote the efficient use of resources in the delivery of community services to elderly and disabled people. Necessarily the focus of attention is on the agency perspective. In particular, local authorities are encouraged to facilitate the provision of services by the private and voluntary sectors. In the field of residential care, financial advantages are to be built in to encourage the reduction in the numbers of establishments directly managed by the local authorities. At the time of writing, the intention is that board-and-lodging allowances are to be paid by the Department of Social Security only for residents in the independent sector; local authorities will be responsible for these expenses in homes that they manage. Several observers (for example, Harrison et al., 1990) have expressed doubts that the independent sector will be prepared or able to take on the problems presented by people with senile dementia given the expected growth in the prevalence in the condition. It is possible that this pressure on local authorities, together with policies encouraging the closure of psychiatric hospitals (Anderson, 1990), will result in an increasing emphasis on the role of the NHS in providing long-stay nursing home accommodation.

The *National Health Service and Community Care Act 1990* requires local authorities to monitor and register residential facilities using an 'arms-length' inspectorate. These inspectorates have a vital role to play in ensuring the well-being of residents and providing guidance to the managers of independently-run homes. To do this requires a well-developed policy basis grounded in an understanding of the effects of residential care environments on the residents. Moreover, in establishing value for money, local authorities will need to be clear that cost containment does not result in unacceptably low-quality care. The main areas of policy concern in the provision or commissioning of residential care for demented elderly people can be summarised as:

- the physical design of homes;
- the issue of specialist provision;
- staffing;
- the role of the homes in the community;
- and performance reviews and monitoring.

Physical design of homes

The White Paper *Growing Older* (Department of Health and Social Security, 1981) drew attention to the contribution of the design of residential homes to the quality of life of elderly residents. Peace (1986) asserts that the design of homes has reflected two competing interests: the desire to create comfortable environments that embody such notions as privacy and choice, and economic constraints. Recommendations for the size and design of homes have varied over the years (Nuffield Foundation, 1947; Ministry of Health, 1955, 1962, 1973). Current issues focus in particular on the use of designs for group living and the balance between personal and public space.

Group-living designs were proposed as a way of combining larger-scale homes (over 25 beds) with a more domestic 'family group' setting (Korte, 1966; Ministry of Health, 1973). It was suggested that the number of residents in a home should be limited to approximately 40, in groups of about eight (Korte, 1966). The design would group together bedrooms, sitting areas and, in some cases, dining spaces (Ministry of Health, 1973). The proposal was that authorities should experiment with the concept of combining 'affinity' groups likely to be compatible with one another (Ministry of Health, 1973).

The issue of greater personal privacy has arisen more recently (Lipman and Slater, 1977; Willcocks et al., 1982). In particular, a national consumer study (Peace et al., 1982) concentrated on eliciting the views of the residents themselves. This highlighted a number of design objectives which, it was proposed, could improve the quality of life for residents. These findings suggest that future designs would maximise dignity and independence if they used the concept of residential flatlets rather than bedrooms. Norman (1984), on the other hand, found that 'public is popular' and the more open the design of public spaces, the more residents competed for places in preference to their bedsitting rooms.

There have been few policy recommendations about designing accommodation for people with dementia. Wagner (1988), for example, contains only two paragraphs on physical design. A number of architects have produced suggestions or specific guidelines. Lipman and Slater (1976) proposed the use of high-rise blocks. Green (1989) identified issues in the building of multi-purpose centres, and Wightman (1992) discusses design principles in planning residential care facilities in details, from strategic planning to complying with fire regulations. Scottish Action on Dementia (1986) have recommended a set of principles for designing residential environments for demented elderly people. These are based on 'normalisation', 'compensation', 'individualisation' and 'integration into the community'. Sometimes these aims – such as 'normalisation' and 'compensation' – appear to conflict. It is not 'normal' to have large, clear notices on bedroom and WC doors, for example. However, naturalistic methods such as 'redundant cueing' – making a message available through more than one sense or 'organised space as orientation' in which any space has a singular and unambiguous use (Pastalan, 1984) – can help to overcome such conflicting objectives.

Marshall (1992) has drawn on a variety of sources and suggests that there is a growing consensus on many aspects of design for people with orientation difficulties. She suggests that buildings should 'make sense' in domestic ways, being small and local and with different rooms for different purposes. Detailed recommendations are based on the principles of creating clarity ('see and be seen'); providing lots of clues, while reducing disorienting features (controlling stimuli); and providing plenty of space for both residents and staff. The recommendations have been based on the specialist needs of people with orientation difficulties. Often, however, the facilities in which people with dementia are cared for will not be specialist.

Specialism

In planning future provision, an important issue is whether demented residents should be segregated or integrated within ordinary residential establishments. Those in favour of segregated facilities argue that they provide a safe, planned environment and avoid distress caused to alert residents in non-specialist homes (Norman, 1987). Those in favour of integration argue that where there are no difficult behavioural problems, moderately demented residents appear to do well and should not represent a problem to other residents (Evans et al., 1981).

The Wagner review (1988) noted the increased use of specialist units in non-specialist homes. This trend has also been observed in the USA. Ohta and Ohta (1988) found that the purposes of such units were varied. In some cases the welfare of the alert residents in the rest of the facility was of paramount consideration, in others the aim was to concentrate resources and specialist knowledge on the demented residents.

In the UK, attention is still centred on the desirability of specialist homes, rather than units. Wagner recommended that:

> Proper provision must be made for elderly mentally infirm people. This will entail closer cooperation between health and social services. Nursing home-type facilities should be developed in association with existing residential establishments (1988, p.117).

This appears to be a call for increased specialisation in the residential care of demented elderly people. However, it is likely that, in policy and practice, specialist facilities will vary as much as specialist units (Ohta and Ohta, 1988). There is a need for evidence to establish whether specialism *per se* or specific aspects of specialist provision can provide a beneficial environment for people with senile dementia. If there are beneficial aspects, it is important to address to what extent these can be incorporated into non-specialist homes in order to benefit demented residents.

Staffing

Staffing policy issues focus primarily on the role, numbers, status and training of staff. *Home Life* (Centre for Policy on Ageing, 1984) provides guidance on the tasks required and groups of staff which should be considered. Guidance on the assessment of staff requirements appears in *Staffing Ratios in Residential Homes: A Platform for the 1980s* (Residential Care Association, 1980). Wagner (1988) found this dated and in *Home Life* it was pointed out that there was no guidance on staff ratios when caring for elderly people who are not heavily dependent, either physically or mentally. The Wagner Review recommended that residential staffing requirements and deployment of staff in all types of residential care should be re-assessed by the Department of Health.

The problems of low status and morale of those working in the field of residential care have been identified by a number of observers (Booth, 1985; Peace and Willcocks, 1986; Wagner, 1988). The Wagner review regarded as a priority the enhancement of the status of staff and recognition of their importance. To this end it recommended that the grading of care staff as manual staff should cease, their posts be redefined as officers or the professional equivalent, and that integrated pay and employment conditions should be introduced for all social services staff.

With regard to training, Wagner recommended that all senior posts should be filled by staff with a social work qualification and that every establishment should be required to draw up a staff training plan which would be subject to registration and inspection procedures. However, in emphasising the importance of social work and in-service training and the role of health services in the care of elderly mentally infirm people, the appropriate training needs of staff dealing with this particular client group are left unclear.

The role of residential homes in the community

Earlier the 'continuum of care' was referred to as though it was indeed in some way continuous, that residential care represented a step within care in the community. In both policy and practice, however, community and residential services have developed almost entirely separately (Willcocks, 1986). This has led to homes being described as 'socially marooned' in the communities they serve (Townsend, 1981).

Links between the community and the home will depend upon the catchment area the home serves, the degree to which visitors come into the home and the services provided by the home to the local community. Various policy documents (Ministry of Health, 1962; Department of Health and Social Security, 1973, 1977) have advocated locating homes close to the community they serve. This enables the residents to be familiar with the area to which they have moved and facilitates visiting by relatives and friends.

The pressure to provide services for the community from residential establishments has grown in recent years due to an awareness on the part of local authorities that a large proportion of resources for elderly people were being devoted to a very small proportion of the elderly population (Allen, 1986). There has been a call for an increased use of homes as resource centres (Barclay, 1982), particularly in the provision of day and respite care (Allen, 1986).

Respite care is provided primarily to meet the needs of informal carers who carry the bulk of the load of caring for this group of elderly people in the community. This can be provided by relief help in the elderly person's home, but more frequently the elderly person goes to stay in a residential home or hospital for one or two weeks to give the carer a break. This has been found, in combination with the use of day care, to have a beneficial effect on carers (Allen, 1983; Levin et al., 1989), although its efficacy in preventing admission to residential care is in some doubt (Melzer, 1990; Levin et al., 1992).

The concern here, however, is the impact on establishments and their residents of policies which encourage links between the community and residential care facilities. The efficient use of resources and desire to relieve and support carers, while admirable aims, must be balanced against the needs of the residents for whom these resources constitute their home.

Inspection, performance reviews and monitoring

Assessing the effectiveness of establishments in providing good-quality care for their residents is a primary role in the new 'arms-length' inspection units of local authorities. Moreover, Wagner (1988) recommended that a condition of registration should be that each establishment should have a system of self-evaluation and performance review. For these to have the desired effect of raising and maintaining high standards of residential care, it is necessary to have a clear understanding of what constitutes good quality and how this can be assessed.

In providing guidance for local authorities, the Social Services Inspectorate has been concerned with redressing an imbalance in methods of monitoring and inspection which tended in the past to focus on regulatory factors such as building standards, staffing arrangements and record-keeping (Department of Health/Social Services Inspectorate, 1989a, 1989b, 1991). Increasingly the focus is on quality of life, quality of care and quality of management. In identifying basic values of concern: privacy, dignity, independence, choice, rights and fulfilment (Department of Health/Social Services Inspectorate, 1989a) and indicators of these values, the SSI has provided a valuable starting point for local authorities. Putting these into practice, however, is another matter. While there may be no difficulty in agreeing that staff should, for example, enable and support residents in fostering independence, evaluating to what extent this happens in practice as a visitor to the home is not a clear-cut task. There are difficulties in establishing consistency of judgements and definitions across even the most experienced inspectors (Gibbs and Sinclair, 1991).

There are also problems in establishing the appropriateness and weighting of criteria by which residential care establishments should be judged. In reviewing the personal evidence to the Wagner committee, the point was made that for younger physically handicapped people the main benefits of residential care were perceived as greater independence from family and institutions. For alert elderly people, on the other hand, a sense of companionship, affection and a family atmosphere seemed to be the main benefits. The review found this

> emphasises again the seriousness of the lack of any direct evidence about what is important to children, the mentally handicapped and the mentally ill (Wagner, 1988, p.159).

This raises the difficulty of establishing the essential ingredients that any monitoring system – at the individual, establishment or agency levels – should identify in order to lay sufficient emphasis on quality of life for elderly people with senile dementia in residential care.

Conclusion

To realise the Wagner committee recommendation that residential care should be a positive choice and experience for this group, an improved understanding of the effect of the residential care environment is required. The types of provision, under the catch-all phrase 'residential care', vary considerably. There is a need to establish the characteristics of homes that provide the most favourable environment for people with senile dementia. In particular, a greater understanding is needed of the effects of the physical design of homes, specialism, the role the home plays as a community resource and staffing issues on outcomes for these residents. Moreover, if monitoring schemes are to be effective they must link into processes that affect the well-being of residents. The aim must be to establish as far as possible what these links are and how to measure them effectively.

This book reports an empirical investigation into the impact of a variety of homes on a sample of residents with confusional problems. While this cannot answer all the questions raised here, it provides a contribution to the growing body of knowledge in a key area of social care.

2 The research questions and study design

The evidence in the preceding chapter pointed towards an increasing need for services for demented elderly people. The role of residential care is likely to be important for such a highly-dependent client group, yet little is known about the features of residential care that will best meet the needs of confused elderly people. There is an absence both of research on which informed decisions might be based, and a clear policy towards residential care for people with senile dementia. This is of particular importance given the increased emphasis on inspection and the need for self-assessment by homes in which quality of life of residents is a key issue, and raises the questions:

- How can the quality of life of demented elderly residents be measured?
- What affects the quality of life of demented elderly residents?

These are wide-ranging issues and no research exercise can hope to answer either in full. However, it is possible to draw on existing work and on models of behaviour to formulate specific hypotheses to use as a basis for research. In this chapter, a coherent, testable model of the relationship between the resident and the residential care environment is developed, the type of questions within each domain are specified, and the design of an empirical study which addressed these questions is described.

A 'testable' model

In an ideal world, the ultimate output quality of life or welfare of the resident would be measured and related to the presence or absence of specific individual needs, and the degree to which the environment met or conflicted with these needs. Both the relationship between the environmental 'fit' and welfare, and the relationship between specific environmental influences and the incidence of 'fit' would be identified. From such a model it should be possible to establish that, for example, residents with certain characteristics (for example, male and depressed) tend to have a high need for order and will thrive in a home with clearly-defined rules and regulations. However, there are a number of difficulties in measurement and methodology that preclude an empirical investigation of such a model when the issue is the relationship between demented elderly people and their environment.

One major difficulty is assessing the quality of life of demented elderly people. Direct reporting of emotional state or morale is likely to be unreliable, if it is achievable at all. People with dementia are dependent on immediate environmental cues, and measures of welfare determined by interview are more likely to reflect the emotional response of the elderly person to the interview than his or her underlying welfare. Moreover, reliably identifying specific environment-related needs and preferences among alert residents is problematic. Those suffering from senile dementia are even less likely to be able to respond to such abstractions.

These difficulties suggest that models such as the 'production of welfare' approach (Davies and Knapp, 1981; Knapp, 1984) in which the emphasis is on final outcomes are inappropriate when investigating environmental influences. The social ecology model, developed by Lawton (1979) and Moos (1976) among others, is considered more suitable in this context. In this model, the relationship between the individual and his or her environment is represented as two-way and non-deterministic. In formulating the model, however, the emphasis is on the demands that the environment makes of the individual. These demands are termed 'environmental press' and are defined empirically:

> an environmental stimulus or context is seen as having potential demand character for any individual if empirical evidence exists to demonstrate its association with a particular behavioural outcome for any group of individuals (Lawton, 1982, p.39).

While quality of life is not addressed directly, the 'ideal' environmental press is represented as that which results in positive affect and adaptive behaviour. This will depend both on the competence of the individual and on various dimensions of the environment. As these are measurable, to a greater or lesser degree, this is a useful starting point for the development of a model relating quality of life of demented residents to the residential care environment. Moreover, the approach incorporates the environmental docility hypothesis (Lawton, 1982). He states that the lower the competence of the individual, the more liable his or her behaviour is to reflect the influence of environmental forces. Thus, although there may be undue emphasis on the impact of the environment on the individual, this was taken as justified when investigating the relationship of people with reduced cognitive competence and their environment.

The model that has been used in this study is illustrated by Figure 2.1, an adaptation of a framework described by Moos and Lemke (1985) in which the personal and environmental influences are linked to adaptive behaviour by means of cognitive appraisal and coping response. In this approach welfare is assumed to underlie non-medical-based changes in competence and behaviour. While a number of different models can prove valuable when adapted to the evaluation of residential care (for example, Bond et al., 1989), this approach was considered particularly appropriate when investigating the care of people with senile dementia, as the emphasis is on the relationship between the competence of individuals and their environment rather than, for example, the structure and process of residential care.

Figure 2.1
Model of environmental effect

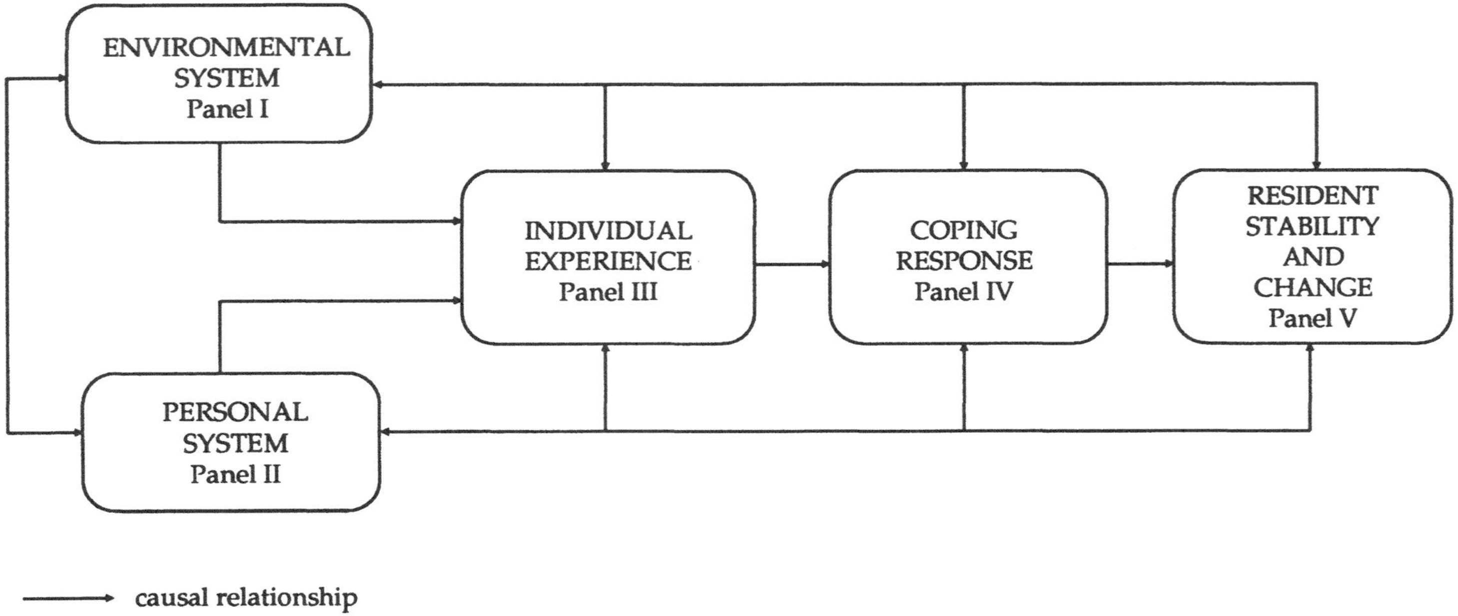

Necessarily the model has been adjusted to permit the inclusion of a set of testable hypotheses for demented elderly people. The principal adaptation that has been made to the social ecology model is that 'individual experience' in Panel III has replaced 'cognitive appraisal' in the original model. While it is not possible to measure reliably what a given experience means to individuals who have senile dementia, it is possible to measure what happens to them. The 'environmental system' in Panel I is thus taken to represent the overall home-level environmental influences (regime, for example) and the 'individual experience', the environmental influences specific to the resident (individual care plans, for example). The 'individual experience' is dependent both on the overall environmental influences and on the personal system, or competences, of the individual.

Lawton (1982) classifies the principal dimensions of the environment as:

- *supra-personal*: the dominant characteristics of individuals in close physical proximity to the subject;
- *personal*: significant others constituting major social relationships;
- *social*: the social climate of norms and expectations; and
- *physical*: non-personal, non-social aspects of the environment.

While the supra-personal, social and physical dimensions are useful distinctions between environmental effects, the adaptation of the model effectively removes the personal environment dimension from the environmental system in the social ecology model. This set of influences is now incorporated in the 'individual experience' of the environment. Thus personal relationships, including visitors, are represented as the individuals' direct experience of the social environment.

In this model the 'coping response' of individuals is distinguished from 'resident stability and change'. The coping response represents the individuals' attempt to adapt either themselves, or the environment, as the result of a specific environmental influence. Thus residents finding their way to where they wish to go will be 'coping' with their 'individual experience' of the physical environment. The individual experience will depend both on the overall design of that environment and on the competence of the individual. Difficulties experienced by residents in finding their way around may result in adaptive behaviour, such as limiting their use of the home to specific areas. Excessive environmental press (such as a particularly confusing lay-out) in relation to an individual's level of competence may result in maladaptive behaviour, such as an increased level of apathy.

This model provides a useful framework for assessing the questions that should be addressed and the assumptions required in assessing the impact of each domain of the environment on demented elderly people. A basic requirement of the empirical design was that there should be clear variation in the environments that residents experience. To ensure that this was so, thirteen different homes were included in the study. The homes were selected to provide a variety of settings rather than a representative sample of residential care facilities. Although a growing proportion of residential facilities are in the private sector, at the time of the study the statutory sector still dominated the provision of residential homes which cater for demented elderly people (Darton and Wright, 1989). Current legislation (*National Health Service and Community Care Act, 1990*) may change this state of affairs so it is important to be clear if any of the results of a study based on local authority provision are unlikely to apply in the independent sector. The problems involved in caring for this group, however, are such that local authorities are likely to continue to play a major part in providing residential care for people with senile dementia (Cox, 1990).

Although the model provides a useful framework, the two-way nature of the person environment relationship poses methodological problems. Everyone acts on their environment to a greater or lesser degree. The degree to which residents have personalised their bedrooms may *reflect* how they feel about being in residential care and/or *affect* how they feel about being in residential care. Great care needs to be taken in deducing causal relationships. For the most part throughout this study, the focus is on how the environment affects the residents. The assumption was that, in so far as they are able, residents have adapted the environment to their needs and observed changes in resident behaviour over time reflect their response to the environment.

From the homes a sample of 104 residents was identified, all of whom had been assessed by senior staff as moderately or severely confused on a four-point scale (mentally alert, mildly confused or forgetful, moderately confused, and severely confused). The homes differed in all the environmental domains of interest. Before specifying these domains, however, it is important to be clear what is required of the measures of outcome and personal characteristics.

Dimensions of outcome and effect

It was not considered practicable in the assessment of demented elderly people to include personal system variables to reflect such aspects as self-concept and personality. In order to make allowance for these, a number of different measures of outcome were included in the model. Each measure of outcome represented an adaptive or maladaptive response. Evidence of maladaptive behaviour can be taken to indicate poor 'fit' with the environment, which can be assumed to be related to a lower quality of life. The type of maladaptive response reflects both the individual and the environment, but enables some inference to be made. For example, if a restrictive regime was associated with higher levels of apathy, it would be possible to infer that demented elderly people who tended to become apathetic would not respond well to a home with this type of regime.

Types of maladaptive behaviour that are associated with dementia include apathy, social disturbance, incontinence and wandering (Gray and Isaacs, 1979). When represented as maladaptive responses to the environment, both wandering and incontinence are particular examples of socially disturbed behaviour. Apathy and socially disturbed behaviour, however, do provide likely alternative reactions to difficult or understimulating situations. While some people might withdraw, others may act in an inappropriate manner or become visibly distressed.

In addition to this it is possible that some environmental influences actively confuse residents. This may not reveal itself in disturbed behaviour but in lower levels of orientation. The many and varied cognitive difficulties (such as memory, information processing and language problems) that may beset a person with dementia have been described elsewhere (Woods and Britton, 1985). 'Orientation' is a general term that refers to an individual's understanding of where they are in time or space. It can be represented as the interface between a person's cognitive capabilities or competence and the environmental demands or press. Too demanding an environment for the individual's competence may lead to confusion or disorientation. Similarly an understimulating environment may lead to deterioration in orientation. Orientation is, therefore, an appropriate basis for a measure of outcome in the model.

There are a large number of scales for assessing the physical, mental and behavioural aspects of elderly people (Kane and Kane, 1981). The requirements of this study were that the assessment should not be too long, should cover all the desired aspects of the elderly person, and establish a suitable basis on which to measure change. For these reasons the Clifton Assessment Procedures for the Elderly (CAPE – Pattie and Gilleard, 1979) were used in assessing the sample residents' abilities and behaviour. These scales have been validated against diagnosis of dementia, concurrently and predictively (Pattie and Gilleard, 1975, 1976, 1978).

The CAPE provided useful subscales for the measurement of these three outcome variables (apathy, social disturbance and orientation). These indicators of behaviour and understanding had the desired property of reflecting the tendency to withdraw or show disturbance. While the scales are perhaps not as long as desirable, this is compensated by the ease of application. This property is not to be minimised as it contributes substantially to the gathering of usable and reliable data.

One further outcome investigated related to the aims and expectations of staff. What do members of staff in a residential establishment work towards when caring for elderly demented people? The aims of policy-makers of 'welfare' or 'quality of life' may be meaningless abstractions for staff working on a day-to-day basis with residents. When care staff are working with people with senile dementia, what are their objectives? A measure of outcome was devised intended to reflect the aims of care staff, based on two questions that were added to the behaviour rating scale (BRS) form of the CAPE. These items reflected the level of agitation and the amount that residents smiled. In the pilot study the officers-in-charge identified these aspects of behaviour as the type of 'output' that they used when monitoring the care of demented residents. The measure derived is represented as an indicator of the contentedness of the residents as judged by senior staff.

It was necessary to measure outcomes over time in order to identify the effect of environmental factors on the resident rather than which types of environment and resident are associated. This latter can reflect policies of admission as much as causal effects. Moreover, to reflect 'resident stability and change', the indicators of outcome needed to measure change in behaviour and orientation over time. Residents were visited at the beginning and the end of a six-month period which was selected as a period that was long enough for change to be observable and short enough for the loss of observations to be minimised. The directions of influence in the model are shown as circular and interactive, but, as discussed above, for estimation purposes and empirical assessment of the hypotheses there need to be assumptions about the directions of causal effects. The period selected was considered sufficiently short to justify the assumption that the environmental system, the individual experience of the environment and the coping response will, given the individual's personal system, effect change in the resident.

There is a major difficulty with using indicators over time as measures of outcome, however. While change over time means that possible bias from selectivity of residents is allowed for, there are inevitably people for whom no information is available at the second stage of the study. This may be because they have died or because they are unavailable for assessment (having been transferred to another home or hospital). In this study there was also one refusal of interview at the second stage (the lady thought the interviewer was from the police). The charge can be made that the results will therefore be biased because there may be a fundamental difference between the survivors and non-survivors.

Table 2.1 shows the destinational outcomes for the sample residents in the study. The assumption made for the current analysis was that over a six-month

Table 2.1
Destinational outcomes

Outcome	Number of residents
Remained at the home	79
Died	18
In hospital – long-term	3
In hospital – short-term	2
Transferred to another home	2
Total	104

period, death and temporary hospitalisation were random events. While this assumption does not hold for permanent transfers to other residential establishments or to hospital, the number of residents who were transferred were very few so this source of bias was limited. An essential element of the analysis, however, is an examination of this potential source of bias (see Chapter 6).

Personal characteristics

In discussing dimensions of outcome and effect it has been identified that some potentially important influences have to be excluded from a testable set of personal characteristics. For example, both attitudes and beliefs are hard to establish but may play a role in a demented resident's behaviour. Snyder et al. (1978) found that residents' life patterns before they entered residential care were an important influence on the tendency to wander. However, Moos (1975) suggested that behaviour outside an institution had little relationship with life inside. The effects of residents' life patterns before they entered residential care may, therefore, have a limited impact on their response to the residential care environment.

Difficulties in adjusting to life changes and stress have been identified as possible influences on the behaviour of demented people (Snyder, 1978; Kirby and Harper, 1988). One of the most important life changes associated with residential care is the impact of the change from life in the community to communal life in a home. A number of studies have found that the process of entry to residential care and the change in environment that results has a deleterious effect on elderly people (Lieberman, 1961; Blenkner, 1967; Markson and Cumming, 1974). There is an increase in mortality and decline in both activity levels and psychological well-being. One explanation of the high mortality rate has been termed the 'relocation effect' (Wittels and Botwinick, 1974).

The potential influences of the relocation effect were excluded by including in the sample only residents who had been in the home for at least six months. The majority of elderly people will have adjusted to residential care after this length of time (Rodstein et al., 1976). While evidence of important personal events during the period of the study was established, stress was represented primarily as the result of poor environmental fit.

The length of time the resident has been in a home is fundamental to the model because this reflects the length of time the resident has been exposed to that environment. Ideally, in the quasi-experimental approach adopted here, outcome measures should monitor all residents from before the point of entry into residential care and follow them through the relocation effect and through to, perhaps, a year after entering residential care. Each resident would then have had an equal 'dose' of the treatment – in this case the residential care environment.

Any such design would have required huge resources to assess properly the large number of homes that would need to be involved, and over the period necessary to distinguish environmental outcomes from the relocation effect. Neither the time nor the necessary resources were available. Different levels of exposure to the environment were allowed for, therefore, by incorporating a measure of length of stay into the model as a control variable.

The competence of residents is fundamental to the ecological model of environmental fit. Physical and mental ability were monitored using the CAPE (Pattie and Gilleard, 1979). However, a resident who is blind or who has a very serious sight impairment will have a very different experience of the environment to other residents. Many of the methods used to communicate with, and assess the abilities of, people with dementia are dependent upon the person being able to see. It was decided, therefore, to exclude those people with serious sight impairments from the study.

Identifying depression in residents is of particular importance because the diagnosis and course of dementia can be fundamentally affected by the incidence of depression (Holden and Woods, 1982; Rabins et al., 1984). It was not possible in this study to draw on a full diagnosis of the condition or assessment of the degree to which behaviour and orientation difficulties of residents were due to depression rather than dementia. When estimating the model, therefore, allowance was made for the effects of depression by adding items to the BRS form which provided indicators of the presence of symptoms of depression and anxiety. These were based on those used by Challis and Davies (1986) who modified the work of Hamilton (1960) in their assessments of community care schemes for elderly people.

Supra-personal environment

In designing the study it was anticipated that much of the variation between homes that was caused by differences in local authority policies and between specialist and non-specialist facilities would largely be captured by variations in specific environmental influences, such as the proportion of confused residents in the home. However, it is possible that some other element, such as higher resource levels generally afforded to specialist facilities, may have an effect on residents that is independent of other individually-measured aspects of the environment. In selecting the sample of homes, therefore, a substantial proportion of specialist facilities were included (six of the thirteen homes). The homes were located in a number of local authorities to reflect a variety of management philosophies in the running of the homes. Five of the homes were located in three outer London boroughs and the remaining eight were sited in a shire county.

In order to provide a description of the resident population of each home, a form based on that used in the PSSRU survey of residential care (Darton, 1983) requesting basic background data and information on disability levels for all residents was sent to each officer-in-charge at the start of the study. This was used as a basis for indicators of the characteristics of the resident population to allow the measurement of hypothesised supra-personal effects. For example, Evans et al. (1981) suggested that in non-specialist accommodation the proportion of elderly people who are 'confused' should not exceed one-third. When there is a higher proportion than this it affects the type of regime and care received by all residents. The information collected about each resident in the home allowed the percentage of confused residents in each home to be included in the analysis.

Staff of the home constitute one of the most expensive and influential aspects of residential care environment. Unlike some of the more intangible aspects of residential care, staffing issues can be directly addressed and influenced by policy. It is all the more important, therefore, that any policy decisions are taken on a properly-informed basis, following research. The foci of interest were actual staffing levels, turnover and training of staff. Staff were asked to complete a questionnaire giving background experience and qualifications, and the levels of sickness and staff turnover were monitored during the study period.

The social environment

Figure 2.1 demonstrates that in the model the individual experience of the environment is dependent both on the environmental system and on the personal system, or competences. This has implications both for hypothesis formation and for measurement of the social environment. For example, the way that rules and normal practice are interpreted for demented residents may differ considerably from the norm in the home. While the majority of residents may be allowed to choose what to wear or to go outside freely, the abilities of a demented resident may be such, or interpreted as such, that these freedoms are perceived as impossible. Thus hypotheses relating to care practices need to specify the expected effects of the home regime and of the individual experience of that regime.

When measuring the dimensions of the social environment, the emphasis was therefore on identifying measures that reflected individual experience as closely as possible. First, a senior member of staff (usually the officer-in-charge) was interviewed to establish the information relating to the overall home caring regime. This included general policies, such as the use of pre-admission visits and care plans, and practice issues, such as the use of set bed-times. Information was also gathered about the number and type of activities organised for residents. In addition, at the beginning of the six-month period a senior member of staff was interviewed to determine how the home's caring regime was applied to each sample resident. This schedule covered: background issues (such as reason for admission), items to assess ability (such as how well the resident could find his or her way around the home), questions about practice (such as the way specific behaviours were dealt with) and other related issues (such as the frequency and types of activity the resident engaged in). This enables the identification of how the social and caring regime of the home actually applied to the resident.

In establishing the broader picture of the social character of the home, measures of social climate should reflect the atmosphere affecting the resident as closely as possible, allowing such questions to be addressed as whether, in a home designed for group living, the social atmosphere varies from group to group. If so, the social atmosphere in an individual resident's group might be of more importance than the overall home atmosphere. Moreover, in non-specialist homes designed for communal living it has been found that 'confused' residents sometimes form an identifiable subpopulation (Harris et al., 1977). This group tends to eat separately and to sit in one or two lounges which 'alert' residents do not use. Where these subpopulations exist, do they form such separate groups that there is an identifiably different social climate among them? If so, the social climate measures used in assessing the effect of the social environment should reflect this.

In establishing the different aspects of the social environment that need to be investigated, use was also made of the dimensions adopted in Moos and Lemke's (1992) Sheltered Care Environment Scale (SCES) (see Table 4.1). This scale forms part of the Multiphasic Environmental Assessment Procedure (MEAP) which was developed from large-scale studies of sheltered care settings for elderly people in the USA. It has been extensively tested and a body of USA-based normative data is available. Some members of staff were asked to complete these for specific groups of residents in order to reflect the hypothesised variations in social climate between groups in group homes and residents with physical, as opposed to mental, disabilities in non-specialist communal homes.

The physical environment

The design of homes for elderly people was identified in Chapter 1 as an important policy issue. Very little evidence appears to exist about the relationship between the physical environment and people with senile dementia. A major obstacle to describing the physical environment is that there is no systematic means of representing information in a way that allows comparisons across different buildings (Keen, 1989).

One of the principal difficulties in designing an appropriate physical environment in which to provide residential care for elderly demented people is the variety of needs that it should fulfil. Ideally the home should combine a prosthetic function with a homely atmosphere (Calkins, 1988). The difficulties encountered by both physically and mentally disabled people should be allowed for, together with the needs for privacy and territoriality. De Long argues that environmental design for elderly people should provide:

> a prosthetic environment to increase the competence of the older person, or an environment reduced in complexity and so clearly encoded that additional redundancy compensates for decreased competence (De Long, 1974, p.108).

Scottish Action on Dementia (1986) also took as a main point of principle that the physical environment should be 'compensating' for disability. This emphasis on compensation fits well into the ecological approach adopted here, but still begs the question of what people with senile dementia as a group require from their physical environment. In establishing these requirements the issue of specialist or non-specialist provision is also raised: are the design needs of people with cognitive difficulties and those with physical disabilities compatible?

The first task is to establish those aspects of the physical environment which are likely to have a particularly important influence in the residential care of demented elderly people. Clearly the physical environment provides warmth and shelter, but the focus here is on the particular needs of people with dementia. Orientation difficulties resulting from the condition mean that such residents will be particularly dependent on external cues, and these cues will not have the long-standing familiarity of those in their own homes. Thus, the degree to which the physical environment provides an appropriate level of mental and physical stimulation, allows socialising and privacy, and facilitates activities of daily living will depend on the degree to which it compensates for the particular difficulties encountered by people with dementia. Three particular aspects of the physical environment suggested by the literature are: the ambience in terms of light and noise (Feier and Leight, 1981); availability and stability of personal territory (Keen, 1989); and how easily residents are able to find their way around (Calkin, 1989).

A rating scale adapted from the MEAP (Moos and Lemke, 1984) was used to assess light and noise levels in the home as well as general comfort and the use of orientation aids. The sample residents' bedrooms were rated individually as indicators of personal territory and the floor plans of the homes were used to assess the overall complexity of the designs and the individuals' experience of them. In addition, assessing the effect of the complexity of the design on residents proved to be one area in which it was possible to estimate a 'coping response', by estimating how well residents could find their way around. The details of the assessment of the physical environment are described in Chapter 5.

Conclusion

Any attempt to assess environmental impact, on demented elderly people in particular, involves compromises and exclusions of potentially important effects. However, the model provides a useful framework for identifying hypotheses and issues in assessing environmental influences. There are pragmatic reasons for the exclusion from the empirical study of many of the 'coping responses', but the use of individual environmental effects and a variety of outcome measures may allow inferences to be drawn about these.

In the following section the results of this study are described. The elements of the social and physical environment are explored in some detail before a model relating these to outcomes for residents is described in Chapter 6. The final chapter discusses these results in the current policy context and the implications for innovative schemes for the care of people with dementia in the future.

3 The social environment: caring regimes

From very early on in the study of residential care of the elderly, there has been a conviction among researchers, observers and practitioners alike that the social environment of homes must have a major effect on the quality of life of the residents. This is demonstrated by approaches such as Barton's (1966) study of institutional neurosis and Goffman's 'total institutions' (1961). The underlying assumption in both cases is that the institutional nature of many homes will have a profound effect on their residents. However, identifying the regimes or social effects of the homes has proved an elusive task. Booth (1985) identified four sets of problems in relating measures of regime to outcomes:

> problems of selective intake; interaction effects between residents and their social environment; the many-sided nature of institutional regimes; and the difficulties of measuring outcomes.

These problems are closely related, especially in the assessment of the effect of the environment on demented residents. The many-sided nature of institutional regimes results in part from the variation in the way that these regimes interact with different groups of residents. Harris and Lipman (1980) suggested that there was a distinction in the way that demented residents were treated both by staff and other residents in non-specialist homes: they were more likely to be found in the least favoured part of a communal area, for example. It was seen as particularly important, therefore, not only to assess the overall regime of the homes but the 'individual experience' of these regimes.

Given the difficulty of assessment, it was decided to take two approaches to the problem of measuring the social environment. These consisted of a set of regime indicators and the Sheltered Care Environment Scale developed by Moos and Lemke (1984). This chapter assesses the first of these, a method based on an approach used by Booth (1985) in which officers-in-charge or senior members of staff were asked about specific management routines and care practices. The advantage of this type of approach was that for many of the questions asked about the general running of the home it was also possible to apply them directly to the individual residents, and see how that particular regime item applied. The disadvantage was in the lack of well-verified scales.

Methodology

Account was taken both of previous studies of residential care and of the specific needs of people with senile dementia when defining the dimensions of the social environment. For example, Booth (1985) identified 'integration into the community' as an aspect of the social environment. In this study, maintaining links with demented elderly residents' backgrounds, or continuity, was considered the most important aspect of such links. Links with the background of residents can provide cues for the residents and guides to appropriate responses from staff (Feil, 1985).

Moos and Lemke (1985) have identified three main dimensions of the social environment: relationships; personal growth; and system maintenance and change. Management routines and care practices were also classified in this way.

Relationships

- *Integration*: the degree to which the residents are integrated into the life of the home.
- *Privacy*: the degree to which residents are able to be separate from the community or 'reserved' (Pastalan, 1978).

Personal growth

- *Stimulation*: the degree to which residents are kept active and participating.
- *Freedom*: the degree to which residents are free to use the facilities of the home and leave the home.
- *Continuity*: the degree to which staff in the home have information on the residents' life history and links that are maintained with the past.

System maintenance and change

- *Planned care*: the degree to which care plans or policies are thought through and discussed.
- *Regimentation*: the degree to which care tasks take place at the convenience of staff rather than the individual needs/desires of residents.
- *Control*: the degree to which residents have control over their lives.

The intention was to devise scales that would reflect the regimes of the homes via management and care practice questions. Since similar questions could be asked at the home and individual level, the scales would demonstrate how the home rating, in terms of regimentation of care for example, related to the actual practice for a particular resident. This was of particular importance in assessing the effect of such factors on demented residents, as their behaviour is often such that 'normal' practice or rules will be seen as irrelevant.

The individual items or questions were selected on the basis of questions used in previous research where it was possible to identify them (King et al., 1971; Evans et al., 1981; Booth, 1985). A detailed examination of the responses in the study to these questions suggested, however, that any scales derived would have been of questionable validity. Once unreliable and invariant items had been eliminated there were insufficient items to provide useful scales of all the dimensions of the social environment that were hypothesised to affect residents. Both in the analysis reported in Chapter 6 and in the following sections, therefore, the emphasis is on responses to individual indicators.

Relationships

The measures were intended to reflect how well demented residents as a whole and individual sample residents were integrated into the home community. There was also a need to assess the positive side of being separate from that community, reflected in the degree of privacy allowed.

Integration

How well integrated a resident is into the life of the home generally will depend partly on the type of home. While the tendency for demented residents to form a separate population in non-specialist homes has been well documented (Harris et al., 1977) and to be 'loners' (Retsinas and Garrity, 1985), it has not been possible to distinguish whether or not this usually is by choice. In practice, the measurement of the degree of integration of residents into the home community proved difficult to establish. It was anticipated that in some homes the more confused residents might be rejected by other residents and segregated by staff. The 'individual experience' of such an atmosphere would be isolation and lack of friendships within the home. However, the items relating to the segregation of the more confused residents proved inapplicable in group-living homes and hard to establish in specialist homes.

In only one of the seven non-specialist homes, five of which were designed for communal living, was there a lounge used primarily by confused residents. In only two of these homes did most of the demented residents eat separately from the alert residents. However, when asked about the attitude of the alert residents to the confused, alert residents were reported as 'accepting' in none of the homes. In two of the homes they appeared to tolerate the confused residents but in four they were rejecting and in one openly antagonistic.

Wilkin and Hughes (1987), in discussing the results of previous research (Evans et al., 1981), suggested that the attitude of alert residents to demented residents in non-specialist homes is dependent, in part, on the proportion of residents who are confused. In this study, the home in which alert residents were openly antagonistic had only 5 per cent of residents moderately or severely confused. Of the two 'tolerant' homes, one had approximately 5 per cent demented residents and the other, 41 per cent. In the remaining non-specialist homes, 20 per cent of residents were assessed as moderately or severely confused. Thus, there appeared to be no relationship in this study between the attitudes of the alert residents and the proportion of residents who were demented.

One of the most important influences on the welfare of elderly people generally is the existence of a confidante or close relationship (Berkman and Syme, 1979). Whether this result holds for people with senile dementia, who tend to have difficulty in forming and maintaining relationships, is less clear. In the social ecology model used here, a 'coping response' to the social environment is the degree to which friendships and relationships are formed and maintained by an individual. This is not easily distinguished from the 'individual experience' of having a confidante or friend. For demented elderly people even this latter is not easily established. In the absence of observational techniques, the assessment of this aspect of individual environmental influence was based on information about observed friendships reported by staff.

On an individual resident level, staff were asked whether each sample resident had a special friend among the other residents, or a special relationship with any member of staff. Of the sample, 36 per cent had a particular resident or couple of other residents with whom they associated on a regular basis. Respondents were often doubtful, however, about the quality of this relationship. If the relationship was of significance to the residents it might be expected that the death or departure of the friend would have a noticeable impact on them. In the six cases where this occurred during the six month period of the study, staff reported no obvious reactions to the absence of the friend.

Friendships with staff were reported less frequently: 27 per cent of the sample residents were reported as having a special relationship with a member of staff. It was more often reported that the resident 'got on' with everybody. Again there was some doubt about what form the special relationships with staff took. In some homes there was an automatic assumption that, if the resident had a keyworker, they had a special relationship with that member of staff. In such cases it was established as far as possible whether this relationship did seem to mean something to the resident concerned.

The converse was also considered and it was asked whether the sample residents had particular enemies among the other residents or the staff. A poor relationship with one or more of the other residents was reported in only fifteen cases. Bad relationships with members of staff appeared to occur even less frequently. Only 6 per cent of residents were reported to be actively antagonistic to one or more particular members of staff.

Privacy

The positive side of a sense of being separate from the community in which a resident lives is the right to privacy. Privacy and territory are often discussed as aspects of the physical environment (for example, Willcocks et al., 1987). Many studies (Kahana, 1982; Booth, 1985; Fyvie and Gledhill, 1989) have defined the provision or allowance of privacy as an aspect of the social environment. The need for privacy is defined in these as a need to be separate from others. Pastalan (1978) described this type of privacy as reserve, associated with the need that people have to withhold certain aspects of themselves. While it is acknowledged that there are physical as well as social aspects to both privacy and territory, here privacy is treated as primarily an aspect of the social environment and territory as an aspect of the physical environment.

While members of staff may respect the privacy of residents who are alert, they may be less careful of the privacy of a demented resident because of fears of 'what they are up to'. Thus the normal practices in a home may be disregarded in what is seen as the resident's own interest. It is important, therefore, to identify as far as possible the degree to which the individual resident is able to experience privacy.

In six of the homes there were facilities for receiving visitors in private. Bedrooms were used in all the other homes. Sixty-one per cent of residents had single rooms and only 9 per cent shared with more than one other resident. Only in five cases did residents share a bedroom in a home that did not have specific facilities to allow them to receive visitors in private. Opportunities for privacy in this respect, therefore, were widespread. However, other aspects of privacy were less well catered for.

Booth found that only about a quarter of homes for elderly people had facilities for allowing residents to lock their rooms. Even where there were facilities, few residents were allowed to hold keys. In the study reported here, just one of the homes, Chaucer Place, had any lockable bedrooms. In this home four of the ten sample residents were allowed to lock their rooms. It is interesting to note that the sole home that catered for this level of privacy was a specialist home and that, in the context of Booth's finding, a relatively high proportion of the sample residents were able to lock their doors. In Booth's study 25 per cent of homes provided residents with a lockable drawer or cupboard. An equivalent number (three) of the study homes allowed the majority of residents a locker of some sort. However, just nineteen of the sample residents overall were actually allowed such a facility.

Personal growth

Personal growth is frequently not an expectation of elderly people in residential care. This is particularly the case in the care of demented elderly people. However, programmes such as reality orientation have shown there is a capacity for improved functioning in specific areas (Holden and Woods, 1982).

The level of stimulation the residents receive is hypothesised to be among the care practices that will encourage personal growth. Both communal activities provided by the home and individual 'rates' of activity will give an indication of the level of stimulation. The degree of freedom that residents are allowed is also represented as an important element of personal growth. Continuity with the past is hypothesised to provide a prerequisite to personal growth for people with the specific difficulties resulting from senile dementia.

Stimulation

The level of organised activities in the home may have a positive, stimulating, effect (Kushlick and Blunden, 1974) on residents or a negative, confusing, effect if they are prevented from withdrawing (Cummings et al., 1972). This will not simply depend on the level of activities or 'stimulation' in the environment; it will also depend on the level of participation of the residents themselves. Thus both the overall level of activities and the 'individual experience' of these, or rate of participation in activities, need to be identified.

The most frequently-organised types of activity were group therapy, clubs, and live entertainment by staff. There was a good deal of variation between the level of activities in homes; from one home that had 48 activities each month (including a daily group therapy session) to a home that had less than one activity each month. It was interesting to note that the high correlation between organised activities and the proportion of confused residents in the home found in the Cheshire study (Kimbell et al., 1974) was also found in these thirteen homes. This was reflected to some extent in the difference between specialist and non-specialist homes. Specialist homes had a higher rate of organised activity (nineteen per month) compared to non-specialist (eleven per month) but the difference was not statistically significant.

Table 3.1 shows that, as would be expected, when the activities organised and participated in are translated into monthly 'rates' there is a high level of correlation between the amount the home organises and the amount the resident experiences. The individual rate of activity excluded reading and watching television as there was often doubt that the resident was registering the television or reading material. Table 3.1 shows a summary of the number of residents who participate and the average monthly frequency by type of activity.

Table 3.1
Activity rates

	Participating residents	
	Number of residents (104)	**Average monthly rate (15*)**
Group-based activities		
Home outings	81	>0
Church service in home	45	2
Music and movement/dance	33	3
Day outings	30	1
Other physical exercise	32	4
Group therapy	22	17
Home clubs	18	6
Church	12	2
Outside clubs	6	5
Individual activities		
Hairdressing	94	2
Watching TV	80	25
Reading	41	23
Sewing/knitting	18	11
Playing cards/games	18	3
Craftwork	10	3
Jigsaws	6	3
House plants	5	3
Gardening	2	2

* Average rate of participation in any activity excluding watching TV and reading.

Residents in specialist homes tended to participate in activities more frequently. The average monthly rate of activity among sample residents was twelve in non-specialist homes and seventeen in specialist homes. There were more clubs in non-specialist homes, and more group therapy sessions in specialist homes. On average the fifteen sample residents who attended group therapy in specialist homes participated 21 times per month while the seven residents in non-specialist homes attended group therapy only eight times each month. Home clubs were attended by eighteen residents in all, approximately once each week, but the seven residents in specialist homes who attended home clubs did so only once each month on average.

The activity which was most regular for most residents was hairdressing. This occurred fortnightly, on average, for 94 of the residents. This usually involved a professional hairdresser visiting the home and took place in a room designed for the purpose. It was included as an activity rather than a personal care task because it involved physical and personal contact in a social rather than a personal care setting. In general, however, there was a low level of individual activity among the sample residents. As mentioned earlier, 'reading' and 'watching TV' were rather dubious categories. Only eighteen residents did any sewing or knitting on a regular basis, ten took part in any craftwork and just two residents took part in gardening.

A 'coping response' that reflects the personal growth dimension is the level of engagement of the resident. The level of engagement of demented people has often been taken as an appropriate measure of outcome in studies concerned with the effect of, or encouragement of, organised activities (Felce and Jenkins, 1979; McCormack and Whitehead, 1981). However, to measure this effectively requires a detailed observational study, which was not possible given the available resources. The assumption was made therefore that a higher 'rate' of reported activity will reflect both the individual experience of the environment and the level of engagement.

Freedom

Another important aspect of personal growth is the level of freedom residents are allowed. A conflicting concern in the care of demented people, however, is safety. Physical and mental dependency upon others may often be the principal reason for admission to residential care (Neill et al., 1988). In fact, too much monitoring may inhibit personal growth by restricting freedom and movement (Clough, 1981). The conflict between a policy of encouraging personal freedom among residents and concern over the safety of a resident with cognitive difficulties may be resolved either by restricting individual freedom or by taking risks. Thus a confused resident's 'individual experience' of a home may differ considerably from another resident's in the same home. It is important, therefore, to determine how restrictions on freedom apply to individual residents.

One home (Viking Lodge) reported that residents were not allowed in their rooms for any part of the day, but in practice none of the sample residents in this home was restricted at all in their use of their bedroom. In fact one resident rarely left it. This is an example where the irrelevance of the home policies to this type of resident results in more rather than less freedom. In the other homes, however, where officially no restrictions on the use of bedrooms prevailed, five of the sample residents were not allowed to use their bedrooms during the day. This reflected the more general case that the concerns of care staff about demented residents' behaviour resulted in more, rather than fewer, restrictions. Similarly, only three residents in the whole sample were restricted from using any of the communal areas in the homes. The one home that reported that there were restrictions on use of communal space imposed no restrictions on two of the three sample residents in the home.

All homes reported that residents were normally allowed free access to the grounds. This reflected Booth's finding that 94 per cent of homes allowed free use of the grounds. However, in practice only 27 per cent of the sample were allowed outside unaccompanied. Although all the homes had gardens, only four of the thirteen homes had an outside area that was enclosed and secure. The lack of a secure area may result in unnecessary restrictions on 'confused' residents because of staff concerns that they might 'wander off' and get lost.

General restrictions on leaving the home unsupervised were confined to five of the homes, all specialist. In fact, however, few of the sample residents were allowed to leave the home freely. Of the six residents who did, four were from homes that specifically did not allow residents to leave the home unaccompanied, providing another example of how the normal rules are often found inapplicable to some demented residents.

It is clear from these items that much of the information collected about home rules and practices have little relevance in practice to the experience of residents who have senile dementia. The level of freedom allowed these residents will depend primarily on perceptions about the residents' competence. How competent residents are perceived to be will depend both on residents' abilities and on the approach of the home.

Continuity

One other aspect of the caring regime that can be considered under the heading of personal growth is the level of knowledge about residents' backgrounds. The previous occupations and habits of demented people may affect the way they respond to stress (Snyder et al., 1978). The greater the understanding which care staff have of the individual and his or her history, the better able they are to understand and respond effectively (Feil, 1985). Such knowledge will depend both on the home's policy on obtaining background information on residents, and on the information and links with the past that exist for the individual. This aspect of personal growth, therefore, also needs to be assessed at the level of individual experience.

Retention of the same GP was included as evidence of continuity of health care and a link with the past. In fact, whether or not residents keep their own GP tends to reflect the type of home: specialist or non-specialist. In all of the six specialist homes less than 25 per cent of residents were estimated to have retained their own GP. The home policy affected the individual experience of the demented residents: of the sample residents in homes where most residents changed their GP, only 10 per cent still had the same one. In homes where about 50 per cent or more were estimated to have kept their GP, 58 per cent of the sample had done so.

Personal possessions acquired over a lifetime form another link with the past, and staff were asked whether residents were allowed to bring in items of furniture. In eight of the homes they were allowed to bring in any items that could be fitted in. This restriction meant that very little furniture brought in by residents was actually in evidence.

The only links with previous background measured on an individual level were in terms of personal relationships. The vast majority (70 per cent) of residents in the study homes received visitors at least once each month, higher than in the PSSRU survey (65 per cent) (Darton, 1986b). However, the sample residents tended to receive visitors less often than other residents in the study homes, with only 64 per cent receiving them at least monthly. This is not entirely surprising as dementia often results in people failing to recognise, or being abusive, to close relatives. Such behaviour is likely to deter even the most devoted visitor. Of the sample residents very few went out with relatives or friends: only 11 per cent went out with relatives at least once a month. Holidays and weekends away were even more rare – just 3 per cent of the residents ever went away.

System maintenance and change

A residential community necessarily requires a level of control and regulation to maintain the running of the home and to introduce and implement changes in the system. This can have both positive and negative effects. On the positive side, planned care can provide a degree of monitoring and response to changes in individual residents' needs that would be impossible in the community. On the negative side, caring for a large number of people with disabilities can lead to regimentation of care practices and a lack of response to individual needs. An important element is the level of control the resident exerts over his or her own life. This may require fine judgement given the nature of the disabilities associated with senile dementia.

Planned care

There is a tendency, perhaps because of the concept of the 'total' institution (Goffman, 1961), to regard a high level of organisation as a negative feature of homes. This need not necessarily be the case in the care of demented elderly people (Ohta and Ohta, 1988). Where residents are restricted in their ability to order their own environment, it may be that a high degree of organisational clarity is a positive influence. For example, the use and implementation of care plans and reviews might reflect an organised, coherent, 'planned' approach to care. To be effective, plans and reviews need to be specific to the individual's needs, so it is important to identify the 'individual experience' of these as well as the use of care plans in the home as a whole.

In eleven of the homes residents normally had a pre-admission visit. In the other two this was rare in practice, however desirable in theory. Of the sample residents for whom there was information, three-quarters had a pre-admission visit. In seven cases the resident had been in the home for so long that this information was not available.

A small minority (ten) of the sample residents had no care plan, policy or general idea to guide care staff, but four of these residents were in a home that claimed to have a formal care plan for all residents! Sixteen residents in all had formal plans and 40 a specific policy. Frequently the latter appeared to have grown from a pragmatic assessment by care staff of the approach that worked best, rather than any coherent policy with expressed aims.

Regimentation

A very rigid approach to organisation may result in a home being less able to tolerate 'challenging' behaviour and deal with it effectively, or in the encouragement of institutionalised behaviour (Tobin and Lieberman, 1976). A rigid task-centred approach to organisation could be reflected in routinisation and regimentation of care practices (Evans et al., 1981). Booth (1985) found that the more dependent residents were usually more tightly regimented than other residents because more caring tasks were associated with them. Thus there may be a considerable difference in the degree to which the home as a whole operates in this way, and the way this applies to individual residents with dementia.

The regimentation indicators used measured the degree to which the personal care tasks, in particular, were geared to the convenience of staff rather than individual residents. On this basis 'block toileting' – that is, regular toileting of residents at set times rather than individually – was an appropriate question at home level but not at an individual resident level. On an individual level toileting may be geared to the staff or residents' convenience but observation would be needed to determine this reliably. In eight of the homes block toileting was reported. Overall, 85 per cent of the sample residents who were incontinent were toileted regularly.

In Booth's study 28 per cent of the homes reported that 'getting up' policy depended on the type of resident. In this study ten homes reported that set getting up times and bathing times determined by staff were the norm. In practice, *all* of the sample residents were woken and bathed at times determined by staff. Neither did anyone have the choice over whom would bathe them, although attempts were made to use keyworkers whenever possible.

Only one home reported that all or most residents were taken to bed at a certain time. A third of the sample residents in the homes where bedtimes were not normally set by staff were put to bed at times set by staff. In Booth's study 61 per cent of the homes reported that whether residents had a set bedtime depended upon their capability. It would seem from this investigation that of prime importance among demented residents was their ability at finding their way around the home. Using a measure described in Chapter 5, those residents who had a set bedtime scored significantly lower on their ability to find their way around, compared with those who went to bed when they chose.

Control

It is also desirable to establish to what extent residents have control over their lives. While it is possible to envisage a situation in which too much choice might serve to confuse a demented elderly person, it is far more likely that the encouragement of a sense of control will serve to enhance orientation. Certainly most studies of outcome measures have found a high association between locus of control and quality of life for elderly people in general (Kuypers, 1972; Palmore and Luikhert, 1972; Challis, 1981).

One of the items chosen to reflect the degree of control residents had over their lives was the existence of a residents' committee. Only one home had a committee although two others reported having tried this in the past. Aspects of daily living that are taken for granted when living in private households are often subject to restrictions in residential establishments. Choice over when or what to eat, for example, or freedom to use the telephone; to choose when and whom to ring. Only two of the homes allowed a regular choice of menu. Eleven of the homes had a pay telephone available for residents, but none had extensions in the residents' bedrooms. It was noticeable that while care may have been taken to install a telephone at such a height that it could be used by a person in a wheelchair, the telephones were often located in very public places, restricting the possibility of having a private conversation.

In all the homes residents were allowed to choose new clothes as a general rule. In practice, however, 29 per cent of the sample residents had new clothes selected for them. Similarly, in choosing what to wear each day, only in one – specialist – home was it not the normal practice for residents to decide for themselves. In those homes where resident choice was the norm, 35 per cent of the sample residents were allowed to decide what to wear in practice.

Conclusion

The indicators of regime provide a useful basis to contrast the individual treatment of residents with dementia with home policies. It is clear from these results, however, that scales based on questions describing the regimes of the homes would not provide a reliable guide to the experience of the individual. Residents with dementia tend to be the exception rather than the rule even in homes specialising in the care of elderly people with mental health difficulties. Often this tendency is exacerbated by the design of homes. Lack of an enclosed outside area reinforces the staff's tendency to put safety considerations ahead of those of promoting personal growth. This is understandable in caring for people with dementia, but can result in unnecessary restrictions. Similarly, lack of opportunity to enforce privacy (using locks) is understandable given some of the behavioural problems associated with dementia, but in most homes there was a sense of minimising risk rather than exploiting potential for forming relationships, personal growth and control.

While individual care practices – such as whether a resident chooses what he or she wears each day – provide a useful insight into the individual's experience of the social environment, there is still a need to measure the character or social climate of the homes. The next chapter addresses this issue.

4 The social environment: social climate and regime classification

While the importance of caring regimes and their direct impact on residents' lives is not to be minimised, there are other aspects of the social environment which will influence the well-being of residents. Of particular importance is the social climate or atmosphere of a home, which can be depicted as the character or personality of an establishment. Gilleard (1989) suggests that dementia can be represented as loss of a sense of self which has to be replaced in part by the caring process. If this is so, it is more than probable that the character of an institution will dominate outcomes of residential care.

A method of measuring the atmosphere of facilities caring for elderly people is the Sheltered Care Environment Scale developed by Moos et al. (1979). This chapter describes the use of the SCES to assess the social climate of the homes and the results are compared to those for American facilities. A method of assessing the variations of social climate within the homes is discussed. The SCES subscales also are used to provide a classification of regimes, an analysis that has been described elsewhere (Netten, 1991, 1992).

Methodology

The SCES forms a part of the Multiphasic Environmental Assessment Procedure developed by Moos and Lemke (1984). This is a set of instruments designed to measure various aspects of the environment of sheltered care settings: the physical and architectural resources, policy and programme resources, resident and staff resources, as well as the social climate resources assessed by the SCES. This has been developed over a number of years and normative data exist for a wide range of facilities in the USA (Moos and Lemke, 1992). The SCES is divided into seven subscales which are intended to reflect different dimensions of the social climate. These relate to relationships, personal growth, and system maintenance and change. The subscales are described in Table 4.1.

The SCES can be assessed by staff, residents, or both, for any given facility. There is provision for the assessment to reflect the ideal institution, the expected or the actual experience. Each subscale is scored as a percentage of responses to nine bivariate items. For the purposes of the present study, the scale was used to measure the staff assessment of the current social climate in the home. In order to minimise variation that might result from the different

Table 4.1
SCES subscale and dimension descriptions

Relationship dimensions	
1 *Cohesion*	how helpful and supportive staff members are toward residents and how involved and supportive residents are with each other
2 *Conflict*	the extent to which residents express anger and are critical of each other and of the facility
Personal growth dimensions	
3 *Independence*	how self-sufficient residents are encouraged to be in their personal affairs and how much responsibility and self-direction they exercise
4 *Self-disclosure*	the extent to which residents express openly their feelings and personal concerns
System maintenance and change dimensions	
5 *Organisation*	how important order and organisation are in the facility, the extent to which residents know what to expect in their daily routine, and the clarity of rules and procedures
6 *Resident influence*	the extent to which residents can influence the rules and policies of the facility and are free from restrictive regulations
7 *Physical comfort*	the extent to which comfort, privacy, pleasant decor and sensory satisfaction are provided by the physical environment

Source: Moos and Lemke (1992, p.3).

perspective that domestic staff might have on the home, only care and supervisory staff were included.

To provide a full picture of the social climate of the home, the SCES assessment should also be completed by the residents. However, the focus of the study was on demented residents, and there would be problems of reliability if such residents were to complete the questionnaire. The memory failings associated with senile dementia are such that the validity of responses would be questionable given that the questionnaire itself is quite long (63 questions) and many residents would be unlikely to complete it. One option would be to seek the views of alert residents, but in specialist homes it is unlikely that there would be sufficient suitable respondents. Moreover, the model predicts that, because of differences in competences, the social climate experienced by demented residents would be very different from that experienced by alert residents, so the usefulness of this perspective would be limited.

Estimating variations in social climate

The problem of the multiplicity of caring regimes within homes (Booth, 1985) has been discussed elsewhere. Two potential sources of variation in the social climate are an identifiable subpopulation of confused residents in non-specialist homes and the characteristics of different groups in group-living homes. In measuring variation in the social climate within the homes, use was made of results of investigations into the validity and reliability of the SCES. An investigation into the effect of individual characteristics of staff on the assessments that they made found that characteristics such as gender and age added at most 4 per cent to the variance of individual SCES scores (Lemke and Moos, 1987). In addition, statistical analysis, using US data, had indicated that only five staff assessments were needed for a home (Moos and Lemke, 1984). It was decided, therefore, that not all the staff were required to make an assessment of the social climate of the home as a whole. Some staff could consider specific groups of residents and thus provide a picture of the variation of social climate within the homes.

In group-living homes, therefore, each member of staff was asked to consider either a group from which sample residents had been selected or the whole home in considering their replies. The assignment was not random unless there was a specific request to make it so. Ordinarily, to obtain the most informed assessments possible, the members of staff most familiar with a selected group were asked to assess that group.

Where homes were not organised on a group basis and if there was an identifiable subpopulation of demented residents, some staff were asked to consider just the demented residents of the home when replying to the questionnaire. Two of the communal homes were specialist so the division was inappropriate, and in one of the five communal non-specialist homes there was no identifiable subpopulation because the demented residents were well integrated and relatively few in number.

Comparison with USA establishments

In comparing the results with establishments in the USA, the first task was to identify the type of American facility which would provide the most appropriate comparison with UK homes for the elderly. The normative data were based on a number of different types of facility. Of these, the nursing homes (127 facilities) and residential care establishments (55 facilities) appeared to be most closely related to homes for elderly people in this country. These have therefore been used as a basis for comparison with the study data in Table 4.2.

UK homes are smaller on average than both nursing and residential establishments in the USA. On average there were 107 residents in each nursing home and 74 residents in each residential care facility in the American sample (Moos and Lemke, 1984). The largest home in the study had 60 beds. The residents of the study homes were both older (84 on average compared with 78 in both types of American facility) and more likely to be female (81 per cent of the residents in the study homes were women compared with about 67 per cent in the American facilities). Resident dependency was established in MEAP on the basis of a percentage score of functional abilities. For all those tasks for which it was possible (nine out of eleven) a score was assessed for the study homes. This was 61 per cent, compared with 38 per cent for nursing homes and 77 per cent on average for residential facilities. On this basis the abilities of the residents in the study homes lay somewhere between the two types of facility.

The social climate in the UK study homes appeared to lie closer to the nursing homes, although even here there were significant differences in the average subscale scores. Table 4.2 shows that the average scores for the study homes were significantly higher on conflict and resident influence, and lower on cohesion, independence and organisation than the nursing homes. The average score for self-disclosure in the study homes was closer to the nursing homes' average, although the difference was still statistically significant. The scores for physical comfort, however, were identical. A similar pattern emerged in the comparison between USA residential care facilities and the results for the study homes.

Benjamin and Spector (1990a,b) used the MEAP to evaluate four British facilities: two hospital wards and two bungalows in a local authority home. The SCES subscales provided a similar picture to the study homes when contrasting them with USA norms, although the level of cohesion was higher and similar to USA levels and physical comfort was significantly lower, as was self-disclosure. The latter two results probably reflect the inclusion of hospital wards in the sample, but the higher level of cohesion provides an interesting contrast with the results obtained here.

Moos and Lemke (1992) used the concept of a 'home profile' to enable comparison to be made between facilities and different assessments, such as the staff and resident view of the same facility (see Figure 4.1). In addition to a direct comparison of the values of the subscales, this diagrammatic method allows a comparison of the relationships between the subscales.

In contrasting the very different profiles of the USA nursing homes and the UK study homes, it could be hypothesised that lower levels of organisation and higher levels of resident influence result in residents feeling freer to express their emotions and this results in higher conflict in the study homes. What appears of more concern, however, is the lower level of independence, especially given the fact that, in the nursing homes at least, a more dependent population is concerned. This may partly reflect the staffing situation: in the nursing homes where the residents are more dependent there is a far higher staff to resident ratio. In the residential homes, where there is a lower staff

Table 4.2
SCES data comparison with US homes

	Study homes	US residential care	US nursing homes
Facility characteristics			
Size (average no. of residents)	40	74	107
No. of staff per 100 residents	51*	42	71
% female staff	96	76	88
% staff employed for more than one year	82	68	54
Resident characteristics			
Average age	84	78	78
% women	81	66	67
% residents in home more than one year	66	70	60
No. of facilities	13	55	127
No. of staff	121	366	2042

	SCES scales					
	Study homes		*US residential care*		*US nursing homes*	
	Mean	SD	Mean	SD	Mean	SD
Cohesion	52	28	75	14	69	11
Conflict	76	17	49	20	64	12
Independence	26	20	55	15	53	9
Self-disclosure	65	22	60	15	63	10
Organisation	53	26	73	14	60	12
Resident influence	71	21	60	16	60	9
Physical comfort	67	13	80	12	67	12

* This includes all staff as whole time equivalent.

to resident ratio, the functional abilities of the residents are much higher. It may also reflect the characteristics of the residents themselves. As pointed out above, the average age of residents in the study homes was higher and there was a higher proportion of women than in the American facilities.

Social climate among confused residents

Given the different ways that home policies apply in practice to people with dementia (see previous chapter) it is reasonable to suppose that their

Figure 4.1
SCES scales: study homes and US norms

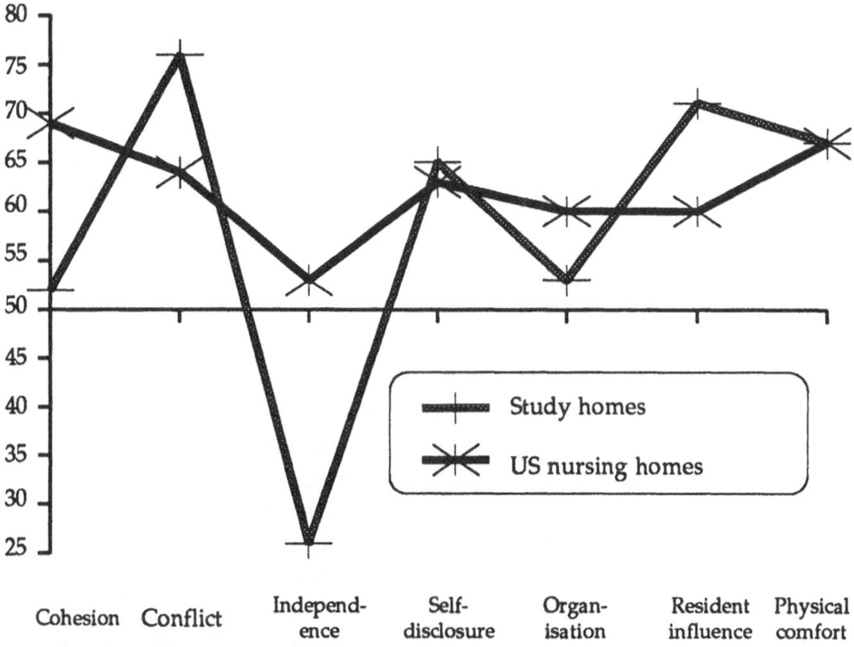

individual experiences of the social climate of residential homes would be different to those of alert residents. The question being addressed here, however, was whether this extended to the social climate among confused residents as a group within each home. For example, do they as a group experience more conflict and less cohesion? The results of the study did not support this hypothesis. When staff considered confused residents for the four homes there was no significant difference on any of the scales from the scores derived from staff considering the home as a whole (see Table 4.3).

The homes were examined separately and again there appeared to be no evidence for a consistently different social climate for confused residents in non-specialised homes. Although the confused residents might form a different subpopulation in some homes, and individual care practices might reflect this, there was no evidence that this extended to a different social climate.

Social climate in group homes

The evidence for identifiable variations in the social climate in different groups in group-living homes was mixed. At the pilot stage the officer-in-charge of

Table 4.3
SCES score for demented subpopulation

	Whole home	Demented residents
Cohesion	36	34
Conflict	71	77
Independence	18	16
Self-disclosure	55	57
Organisation	51	47
Resident influence	63	65
Physical comfort	62	64

Four non-specialist homes were included.

the group-living home considered that the scales did reflect differences in the character of the groups in her home. There were also some examples in the full study of homes where the social climate of the group was clearly different in some respects to the home as a whole. For example, in Viking Lodge one group had a statistically significant higher level of conflict (91) compared to the other group assessed (63). This group appeared to affect the whole home as the conflict score for the home was 85. The level of self-disclosure was also significantly higher in the group with the high level of conflict. In one other home (The Laurels) the level of conflict also varied significantly. In this home, however, there was more conflict in the home as a whole (76) than in the individual groups measured (68 and 47). To establish whether this was due to the influence of a group not included in the study, or perhaps to some conflict between groups, would need further investigation.

Generally, however, there was not much variation within group-living homes between groups in the study homes. There appeared to be very little work towards, or emphasis on, forming a sense of group identity. Moreover, in several of the group-living homes, staff were not allocated to a specific group but rotated between groups. This was in order to be fair to the staff, so no one was constantly allocated to the group that generated the highest workload. Clearly, in such homes the emphasis was on the needs of staff rather than of residents. Such practice and the absence of any policy of developing the groups within the homes suggest that it is unlikely that the family group atmosphere intended (Korte, 1966) is likely to develop.

Groups were more clearly defined both physically and organisationally than subpopulations of confused residents, making assessments by staff more straightforward. The evidence suggests that the SCES subscales were identifying variations in the social climate in group homes, where they occurred. Further work would be needed to confirm this. But while the internal variation in social climate appeared limited, the variation between homes was significant for all dimensions except conflict and physical comfort. This seemed worth exploring in more detail and is discussed further below.

Classification of homes by regime type

The SCES scales provide useful indicators of individual aspects of the social climate and the profiles provide a method to compare types of facility. There is a need, however, for a more general description of the homes, classifying them by regime type or social climate profile, providing both a descriptive device and a tool in further analysis. Timko and Moos (1991) have developed a typology of social climate based on the analysis of a wide range of USA establishments. Using cluster analysis on the results for 235 facilities, they identified six types of social climate: supportive, self-directed; supportive, well organised; open conflict; suppressed conflict; emergent-positive; and unresponsive.

In describing types of regime in British homes, it is useful to refer to three principal types of regime which have been identified in previous research: positive, mixed and restrictive (Booth, 1985). These were described as:

- *Positive*: homes which tend to allow residents to do or decide things for themselves, leaving them a greater area of freedom of action and individual choice.
- *Mixed*: homes with multiple regimes, opportunities for freedom and choice in some areas and not others, and those whose approach consistently falls between the other two groups.
- *Restrictive*: homes that tend to adopt a narrow or restrictive view of residents' capabilities, limiting freedom of action and denying opportunities for deciding things for themselves.

If this basis for describing the regimes is to be used in a classification using the SCES subscales, the most important subscales to be defined clearly are independence and resident influence. With the exception of physical comfort, all the dimensions of the social climate were used to determine the clusters as the subscales are interdependent and reflect other important aspects of the social climate.

Methodology and resulting classification

Cluster analysis (Everitt, 1980) was used as a purely exploratory technique in identifying whether the SCES subscales, based on assessments of the home as a whole, could be used to determine the types of regime.

The clusters were examined when there were two to six clusters inclusive, to see if a pattern could be distinguished. The grouping of the homes at each stage is detailed in Table 4.4. The initial division into two clusters appeared

Table 4.4
Cluster analysis of homes

1	2
Viking Lodge	Pondlea*
The Copse	Haddock Lodge*
Greendale	Chaucer Place*
The Laurels	Westgate*
Victoria House	
Centrelea	
Goldacre†	
Airedale House†	
Thayler House†	

1	2	3
The Copse	Pondlea*	Viking Lodge
Greendale	Haddock Lodge*	
The Laurels	Chaucer Place*	
Victoria House	Westgate*	
Centrelea		
Goldacre†		
Airedale House†		
Thayler House†		

1	2	3	4
The Copse	Pondlea*	Viking Lodge	Chaucer Place*
Greendale	Haddock Lodge*		
The Laurels	Westgate*		
Victoria House			
Centrelea			
Goldacre†			
Airedale House†			
Thayler House†			

1	2	3	4	5
The Copse	Pondlea*	Viking Lodge	Chaucer Place*	Airedale House†
Greendale	Haddock Lodge*			
The Laurels	Westgate*			
Victoria House				
Centrelea				
Goldacre†				
Thayler House†				

1	2	3	4	5	6
The Copse	Pondlea*	Viking Lodge	Chaucer Place*	Airedale House†	Goldacre†
Greendale	Haddock Lodge*				Thayler House†
Victoria House	Westgate*				
Centrelea					
The Laurels					

* Homes classified as having positive regimes
† Homes classified as having restrictive regimes

to divide the homes with positive regimes from 'the rest'. Subsequent clusters, however, did not quickly identify restrictive regimes. Initially, specific homes were identified as having particular individual characteristics.

Viking Lodge formed a separate group once three clusters were identified. Figure 4.2 shows the difference between the SCES profile of this home and the profile given by the average scores of the other homes. Cohesion, organisation, self-disclosure and independence were significantly lower than in the other homes. Conflict was also higher, although the difference was not statistically significant and may have been due to a particular problem in one group. The officer-in-charge left this home during the six months following the assessment. This suggests that the social climate of Viking Lodge was stressed at the time of the assessment and the social climate scores reflected a temporary problem rather than a particular type of home.

The separation of Chaucer Place, once four clusters were identified, into a separate group reflects a difference in the way this positive regime was generated. This home had a very devolved structure, using keyworkers in the decision-making process. Thus the subscale score for organisation was very much lower than in the other positive homes, where the personality of the officer-in-charge appeared to be working to motivate other staff in generating the positive, professional regimes. Although this is obviously of interest, it was felt that the type of regime – higher independence, resident

Figure 4.2
Stressed home versus other homes

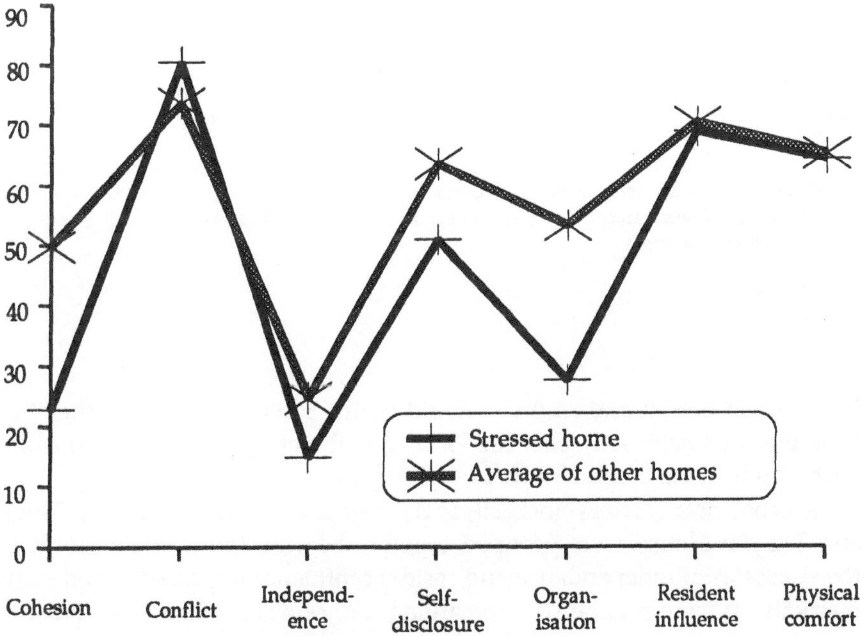

Table 4.5
Distinguishing regime types

	Positive		Mixed		Restrictive	
	Max	Min	Max	Min	Max	Min
	(Mean)		(Mean)		(Mean)	
Cohesion	81.7	55.6	48.9	18.5	51.1	20.6
***	(75.4)		(37.7)		(32.9)	
(51.6)						
Conflict	87.3	71.4	85.2	67.8	75.5	68.9
NS	(77.6)		(75.7)		(72.6)	
(75.8)						
Independence	51.6	31.0	27.2	13.6	10.2	8.9
***	(38.4)		(21.3)		(9.9)	
(25.5)						
Organisation	71.4	46.0	58.9	18.5	51.1	38.4
***	(65.0)		(44.1)		(44.7)	
(52.5)						
Self-disclosure	86.1	60.3	58.3	51.1	56.5	44.4
***	(80.6)		(55.4)		(52.7)	
(64.8)						
Resident influence	90.5	81.7	74.4	56.1	51.4	44.4
***	(85.9)		(68.2)		(48.8)	
(70.9)						
Physical comfort	74.6	55.6	69.1	53.7	76.9	53.3
NS	(68.0)		(64.9)		(66.7)	
(66.7)						

Figures in brackets refer to average scores
Significance levels refer to analysis of variance (F statistic) of scales between regime types

NS $p > .1$
*** $p < .01$

influence, cohesion and so on – should be the principal divide, rather than how this was achieved. Chaucer Place was therefore classified as positive, with Pondlea, Haddock House and Westgate.

No other clear clusters emerged, so the homes of Goldacre, Airedale House and Thayler House were grouped together because the average scores for the subscales of independence and resident influence appeared to reflect the restrictive type of regime. The remaining homes were defined as mixed.

Description of regime groupings

Table 4.5 identifies the average and range of scores in each type of regime. The home classifications vary significantly on all the scales with the exception of physical comfort and conflict.

Figure 4.3 shows that the profile of the homes with positive regimes is clearly different to that of the other types of home. The positive regimes were easily defined using the cluster analysis and have significantly higher resident influence and independence scores, which were identified at the outset as being important if the groupings were to reflect the type of regimes proposed by Booth. Cohesion is much higher in these homes and at a similar level to conflict. Both the levels and the profile of the SCES subscales are closer to the USA profile of nursing homes (Figure 4.1). Independence is lower in the positive homes, however, and resident influence higher than in the American facilities. The profile of positive homes is nearest to the 'emergent-positive' in the typology of climates identified by Timko and Moos (1991).

The homes which had a restrictive regime were not so clearly defined in terms of the cluster analysis, and their profile in Figure 4.3 is less easily distinguished from the homes which were classified as having a mixed regime.

Figure 4.3
Types of regime

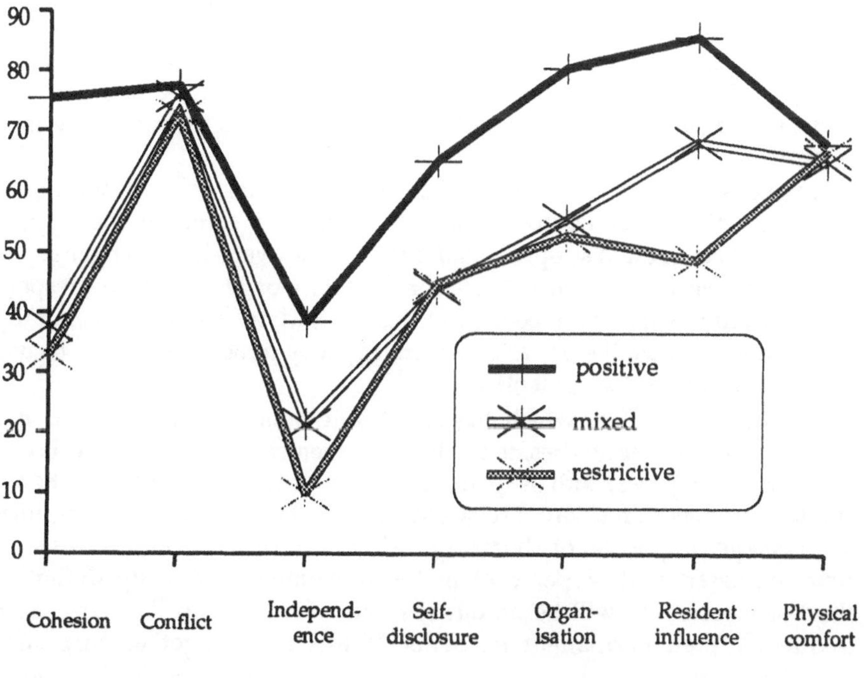

They clearly differ, however, from the other homes on the critical dimensions of independence and resident influence. Both the restrictive and mixed profiles were similar to the 'open conflict' type of home identified by Timko and Moos (1991).

Further work needs to be done over a larger sample of homes to establish both normative levels and measures of concurrent validity. It is interesting to note that the types of climate most closely match the types found to predominate nursing homes in the USA. This analysis provides at least a starting point for developing a usable measure. For example, if the results of the study were validated by further research then one classification would be that a home scoring over 30 for independence *and* over 80 for resident influence could be defined as having a positive regime. If a home scored less than 12 on independence it would be regarded as having a restrictive regime.

Determinants of type of regime

Caution is necessary in drawing conclusions from aspects of the homes which appear to be associated with the type of regime, as most of the data collected are cross-sectional. With such data there is often a lack of clarity about the direction of cause and effect. However, it is interesting to note that both positive and restrictive homes are significantly associated with a higher proportion of confused residents. On average, 18 per cent of residents were assessed as moderately or severely confused in the mixed homes. This compares with 67 per cent of residents in the restrictive homes and 48 per cent in the positive homes. This finding reflects the distribution of the specialist homes. Only one of the six specialist homes fell into the mixed category. Two of the specialist homes were classified as restrictive and the remaining three as positive.

It is possible to speculate that when there is a substantial proportion of residents with dementia, homes have to abandon a commonsense type of regime otherwise often adopted. Staff may become overwhelmed by the sheer quantity of work and their concern for the safety of residents, and respond by restricting them and becoming more rigid in approach generally. Alternatively, a positive professional strategy may be adopted which focuses on maximising resident potential.

Another association which has important policy implications, if it is confirmed in further studies, is the link between short-stay care and homes with positive regimes. Both the percentage of short-stay residents in the homes and the turnover of residents are negatively associated with positive regimes. The average proportion of short-stay residents in positive homes was 1 per cent compared with 4 per cent in the remaining homes. By definition, short-stay residents will be admitted to and depart from the home more frequently than permanent residents. It was not altogether surprising, therefore, that there was a turnover of nearly 100 per cent over a six-month period in the homes of mixed or restrictive regimes. The turnover of residents in the homes with positive regimes was still high (74 per cent), but the difference was statistically significant.

It is probable that the lower level of turnover of residents in homes with positive regimes reflects the proportion of short-stay residents. If there is a causal connection, it is most likely that the resentment expressed by permanent residents towards short-term admissions noted by other observers (Kuh and Boldy, 1981; Allen, 1983) is reflected in the social climate of the homes. If the provision of short-term care by long-term care institutions prevents the formation of positive regimes, this calls seriously into question whether using these homes to provide relief care is appropriate.

This presumes, however, that provision of these positive regimes is an aim of residential care. If these regimes are to be as desirable as the classification of positive would imply, it is necessary to establish a relationship with outcomes for the resident.

Conclusion

Two methods of addressing the problem of measuring the impact of the social environment were adopted. Both in describing the social climate of homes as a whole and in developing a classification of homes, the SCES scales have been successful. The classification was based on Booth's (1984) types of regime and one of the most important distinguishing dimensions was the independence subscale. It is interesting to note that the average score for independence in the homes with a positive regime was still lower than the *average* for both nursing homes and residential care facilities in the USA.

The SCES approach did not distinguish any different social climate for the demented elderly residents as a group in non-specialist homes. However, in homes designed for group living, each group was clearly identifiable by staff. Absence of statistically-significant variation between most groups within homes probably reflects genuine lack of variation between these groups. Where variations do exist, however, they are likely to have a more direct impact on residents than the social climate of the home as a whole. For example, if there is a high level of conflict in a resident's group, it is this, rather than the level of conflict in the home as a whole, which will exert the most effect.

In further analysis, therefore, it was decided to incorporate variables indicating the overall regime type (positive, restrictive or mixed), the SCES scores for the home as a whole in homes designed for communal living, and the SCES scores for the resident's group in homes for group living. These indicators, together with the measures of individual care practice identified in the previous chapter, provide a basis for assessing the impact of the social environment on demented elderly residents.

5 The physical environment

Both indirectly (that is, as an influence on the type of social environment that develops) and directly, the physical environment will affect elderly people's experiences of residential care. As with other aspects of the environment, however, it is important to be aware that even with very reduced competence levels, elderly people with dementia are not simply subject to their environment; they are active participants. Frequently officers-in-charge or matrons of wards tell of schemes in which they try to put the chairs in sitting areas into cosy groups to encourage social interaction, only to find them mysteriously all with their backs to the walls again. This is done not by the cleaning staff, but by the residents: they are not there to socially interact, they are there to keep an eye on things and a chair with its back to the wall is the best way to do that. As with other aspects of the environment, therefore, the emphasis in the study reported here was on individual experiences and the needs of the elderly person.

Three principal dimensions of the physical environment were investigated: ambience, extent of personal territory, and complexity of the environment. After a brief description of the types of design of homes included in the study, this chapter discusses the ambience and extent of personal territory. The main focus, however, is on the complexity of the design as experienced by the sample residents. This is primarily because an attempt was made to measure both the coping response of the sample residents (ability to find their way around) and sample residents' individual experiences of the complexity of the environment. This was first reported in Netten (1989).

Types of design

The homes in the study varied in design from a conversion of a private house to new purpose-built establishments. The majority were constructed relatively recently: five were built since 1980. The building stock was therefore rather younger than that found in the country as a whole in 1981 – only 31 per cent had been built within the ten years preceding the national survey.

Norman (1984) identified four types of residential home design: purpose-built single unit; group unit; ward-like unit; and converted private house. In the empirical investigation, none of the homes was of the ward-like unit type or of the 'race-track' design of the purpose-built single units. Two of the homes were converted private houses, six were designed or adapted for group living and five were of the 'finger' model communal design.

According to the definitions used in the PSSRU survey (Darton, 1986a), only 30 per cent of establishments were classified as group or semi-group-living homes in 1981. The high proportion of group-living homes in the study reflected the policies of the local authorities concerned. One of the homes was in the process of conversion from a former purpose-built home for communal living into a group-living establishment, and plans were underway for conversion of another of the homes to enable group living. Moreover, of the five homes built during the last four years, four were for group living.

The definition of a group-living home for the purposes of the study was one in which the primary activities of daily living, eating and sleeping were confined to a definable area for a particular group of residents. The residents themselves were not confined but did not need to leave the area. Typically such a home would be of dispersed design with two or four dining and sitting rooms. Bedrooms would be in close proximity to these, with WCs and bathrooms nearby. Unless the resident was leaving the building, there would be no need for them ever to visit the rest of the home. Figure 5.1 shows an example of a floor plan of a group home.

Communal homes, on the other hand, were characterised by a single dining area for all residents. There were usually several sitting areas, but the larger communal areas tended to be concentrated in one part of the home, away from the bedrooms. The purpose-built communal homes frequently had long corridors. Figure 5.2 gives an example of a floor plan of this type of home. Only two of the homes in the study were converted from older residential properties. These were classified as communal and could be represented as more normal, or more like private housing, at least on arrival at the home. However, later additions and the scale of the buildings did mean that they had relatively complicated lay-outs. For a visitor to the home, it was generally found easiest to navigate the traditional, communal purpose-built homes.

Residents of homes use the physical environment in a number of different ways, such as for privacy, and for mental and physical stimulation. Above all they use it for activities of daily living. Reduced cognitive competence means that if they are able to use the home, an essential feature of the physical environment is clarity. It needs to be easily understood and make sense to residents with dementia if they are to be able to retain as much independence as possible (Coles et al., 1992). Central to a clearly-understood environment is the ambience of the home.

Ambience

The ambience in this context incorporates the level of lighting and noise in the home. A quiet atmosphere and bright surroundings mean it is easier for a resident with reduced sensory abilities to see and understand what is going on (Feier and Leight, 1981). A coping response to excessive noise or inadequate light may be to change the environment, by going to a quieter place or turning

Figure 5.1
Floor plan of a group home

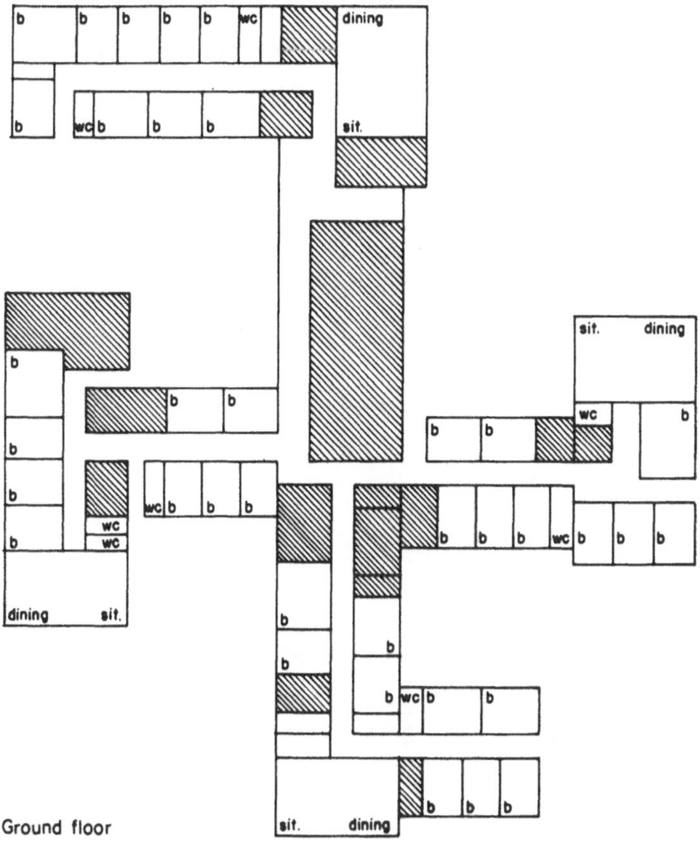

Zones:	Bedroom	6
	Sitting room	4
	Corridor	9
	Total	19

on a light. Where reduced competence or environmental restriction does not allow such coping responses, the result may be social disturbance, withdrawal, or a reduced level of orientation.

A four-point scale from the MEAP Rating Scale (Moos and Lemke, 1984) was used to rate the light and noise levels in the bedrooms, sitting areas, dining areas and corridors. Emphasis was laid on those groups in which residents in the sample spent most time. The scores were added to give two

Figure 5.2
Floor plan of a communal home

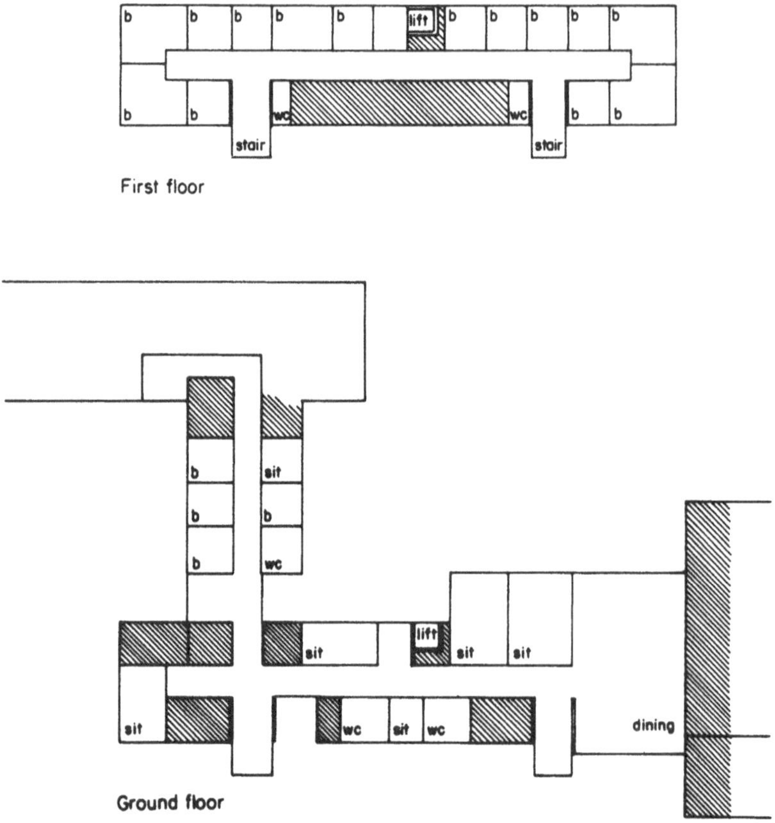

Zones:	Bedroom	2
	Sitting room	6
	Corridor	3
	Total	11

indicators of the overall level of light and noise.

The design of homes directly influenced the lighting levels. Purpose-built communal homes were much lighter overall, due mostly to the level of natural light as they often had large picture windows in sitting areas and along corridors. The darkest home was one of the older buildings that had been converted for use as a local authority home. In general, however, the newer homes designed for group-living were darker, with much less natural light from windows, and with internal corridors dependent on artificial lighting.

Overall the homes were quiet, although in individual sitting rooms the sound of the television sometimes dominated. Other than the television the main source of noise was 'entertainment' (often in the form of very loud music) or the shouts of a demented resident. It is perhaps worth recording what was not evident. There was no quiet music and in none of the homes was there a 'hum' of conversation. This is not to imply that people did not talk to one another, it was simply that such conversations that did occur took the form of isolated remarks, questions and comments.

The level of noise did not appear to be related to any particular design feature in the homes. The physical lay-out, however, was related to the amount of territory or personal space available to residents.

Territory, privacy and personal space

An important aspect of the physical environment is 'defensible space' or territory (Newman, 1972). When people live in private households this takes the form of a house or flat and, depending on the design, some of the surrounding area. This confers status; it is a symbolic token of having a 'stake in the system' (Newman, 1972). Personal space becomes territory if the person has control over that space (Keen, 1989).

It is important to be clear about the distinction between privacy and territory. Keen (1989) distinguishes three dimensions of physical privacy: visual, acoustic and olfactory. Although privacy and territory are very closely-linked aspects of personal space, not all territory will be private on all three of Keen's dimensions. For example, the chair where a resident always sits in a lounge will be a place that they can be seen, heard and smelt! That chair, however, may form an important part of the resident's territory. Similarly, a room which residents may use to receive visitors may afford privacy while not forming part of a resident's territory. In the following discussion 'personal territory' is defined as space that is potentially both private and territorial.

Willcocks et al. (1987) follow others (Lawrence, 1982; Rapoport, 1982) in dividing the physical environment of homes for elderly people into public and private space. In their study public space included lounges, dining rooms and circulation spaces. Private spaces consisted of bedrooms, bathrooms and WCs. The importance of personal territory can be seen by the extent of its use. Stephens and Willems (1979) found that residents in two homes spent an average of two-thirds of their time in their own rooms. The need for adequate personal territory in the design of homes led Willcocks et al. (1987) to recommend that future homes provide residential flatlets rather than the small single and shared bedrooms currently provided.

Although the concept of personal territory primarily relates to the physical environment, there is also an important social dimension. Kellaher (1986) suggests that in residential care physical disability can mean that control over space is restricted to cognitive control. Restrictions on use or constant invasion by staff or other residents will undermine any sense of ownership or personal territory that a room can offer. Necessarily there will be some overlap, therefore, between the social environment factors discussed in earlier chapters and the notion of personal territory.

Establishing territory

The only areas in residential facilities that 'belong' to residents are their bedrooms but for these to provide clearly-defined areas of personal territory they need to be single. Lipman and Harris (1980) found that shared accommodation was disproportionately allocated to confused residents although there are anecdotal reports that suggest many demented residents are happier when sharing a bedroom. A higher incidence of residents with senile dementia sharing bedrooms may reflect the relatively low status of 'confused' residents in non-specialist homes rather than differing needs. This latter theory is supported by the finding that confused residents suffer from being rejected by other residents, even to the point of being pushed out of favoured chairs (Lipman, 1968).

Ten of the thirteen study homes had a maximum of two beds in any bedroom. This compared favourably with homes nationally: in 1981 only 57 per cent had a maximum of two beds in any bedroom (Darton, 1986a). Those homes with the largest number of beds per room were both converted from previous use as private housing. One had a five-bedded room and the other four rooms with four beds each. A purpose-built home for specialist care of mentally infirm elderly people had an unusually high proportion of shared rooms: only six of the nineteen rooms were single. There was provision in the design, however, to convert most, if not all, the shared rooms into single rooms at a later date if desired. There was no evidence of the sample residents disproportionately being allocated shared bedrooms in the study homes: 62 per cent of the beds in the study homes were in single rooms and 61 per cent of the sample residents had single rooms.

Where sample residents shared bedrooms, an attempt was made to assess how clearly-defined was the part of the room that belonged to the resident. Judgements of the arrangement of the furniture and any personal territorial markers were used to make this assessment, rather than observation of behaviour. While there appeared to be no observable division at all for only two residents, none of the residents had part of the room very clearly defined as his or her own. In the majority of cases (59 per cent) there was little observable separation of area.

Much policy and research emphasis has been laid on the size of bedrooms (Ministry of Health, 1973). From the perspective of the individual residents, however, it is the size of their territory that is of importance. The size of residents' territory in this study varied considerably. On average each resident had a bedroom area of 8.95 square metres but the areas ranged from 2.00 to 11.00 square metres. Single rooms were larger on the whole (9.62 square metres) and those residents who had little in the way of identifiable territory markers had smaller areas of territory (7.58 square metres). In 1973, the revised Local Authority Building Note No. 2, recommended that single bedrooms should have a minimum area of 10 square metres and double rooms 15.5 square metres. While the average bedroom area by room type is very close to these recommendations, many of the sample residents have very much smaller areas of territory.

'Personalisation' of rooms, by bringing in furniture and other personal possessions, can be seen as a method of establishing a sense of territory. Personal belongings are important in preserving a sense of identity, and also affect the way people are perceived by other residents and staff. Millard and Smith (1981) showed that elderly people surrounded by personal belongings were perceived in a less negative way than the same people in bare surroundings. Although the general policy of allowing residents to bring personal possessions and furniture into homes is widespread, in practice residents tend to bring in very few things (Norman, 1987).

This was reflected in this study. Residents (or their relatives) rarely individualised bedrooms by bringing in possessions and furniture although most have encouraged the practice (see Chapter 3). Bedrooms provided a limited amount of space but there was little evidence that rooms were being filled as far as possible. Indeed, the rooms which were clearly a separate, personal area in the home were the exception rather than the rule. Only five residents in the sample had personalised their bedroom to any great degree. A further third of the sample residents had personalised the room noticeably. In seven cases there was virtually no evidence of habitation other than standard home-provided furniture and bedding. The majority (56 per cent) had personalised their rooms only a little, with one or two ornaments or pictures.

Residents with dementia clearly need a great deal of support in personalising their territory. In addition to looking for evidence of this positive personalisation, the issue of whether territory was undermined was also investigated.

Undermining territory

Two indicators of the physical environment included were assumed to represent the institution undermining the residents' sense of territory. These were observation windows and change of bedroom. Only in one (new) home were observation windows the norm. These took the form of frosted glass panels from the bedrooms on to the corridor. Although it was not possible to see clearly through these, they gave at least the illusion of an invasion of privacy.

Seven per cent of sample residents who remained in the home at the end of six months had changed their bedroom during the period of the study. The reasons for the change of room were varied: deterioration of residents' behaviour, or deterioration of behaviour in the person with whom they shared; movement of residents into better rooms and so on. However admirable the motive, the result may well be a reduction in continuity of a sense of personal territory for that resident and it was not clear whether this was taken into consideration in such decision-making. The lack of personalisation of the bedrooms may have contributed to the sense in which some of the staff saw bedrooms as a side issue, while for residents they are likely to be central to their experience of residential care.

Own chairs as territory

Insufficient sense of territory may lead to defensive behaviour, or simply a sense of being a constant visitor in his or her own home. One characteristic of some homes is that all, or nearly all, residents always sit in their 'own chair' (Davies and Knapp, 1981). In these 'own chair' homes every resident has a place where they sit which is rarely varied, and is strongly defended if threatened. One explanation is that this is a form of territorial behaviour which dominates certain homes.

In eight of the study homes nearly all the residents sat in their 'own' chair. Of the sample residents, approximately half (47 per cent) always sat in one particular place. As would be expected, this was heavily influenced by the home culture. Seventy-one per cent of the 58 sample residents in the 'own chair' homes always sat in the same place. Only 18 per cent did so of the 45 residents in the remaining homes.

It is interesting to examine this in relation to other indicators of personal territory. Table 5.1 shows the association between homes with the 'own chair' culture and other territorial indicators. The average bedroom area for the sample residents in these homes was significantly lower and, where residents shared rooms, the divide between areas was less well defined on average. Also, the proportion of single bedrooms was lower, although this was not statistically significant.

One possible underlying reason for these relationships is the age of the homes. Once established, the 'own chair' culture, as with the tendency to have all the chairs around the edge of a sitting room, is difficult to change, even if the attempt is made. It is possible that staff used to positively encourage residents to regard one chair as their own in the older homes, even if they no longer do so. Homes built before 1971 have significantly smaller bedroom areas (7.2 square metres) than homes built since (9.5 square metres). In all of the homes built before 1970 the 'own chair' culture dominated. However, of

Table 5.1
Indicators of personal territory

	Type of home		
	'Own chair'	Other	p
Average bedroom area (m^2) (n = 104 residents)	8.33	9.76	***
% of those in shared room where there was little or no divisions (n = 41 residents)	80	38	***
% of bedrooms that are single (n = 12 homes)	52	70	ns

Analysis of variance (F statistic)
ns $p > .1$
*** $p < .01$

the nine homes built since 1970, four had the 'own chair' culture and in these homes the bedroom area was smaller (9.2 square metres on average) than those where the culture did not persist (9.8 square metres).

Without a larger sample of homes and a more detailed study of territorial behaviour, it is impossible to deduce much from these associations. It is of interest, however, that there does seem to an association between this culture of residents having their own chair and the extent of personal territory. The dimension of the physical environment where there was the clearest evidence of a relationship between design and resident behaviour was the analysis of the complexity of the design and residents' ability to find their way around.

Complexity

A major design concern in the care of elderly people with dementia is the need of residents to orientate themselves spatially (Calkin, 1989). Residents need to be able to find their way to where they wish to go if they are to exert even minimal control over the activities of daily living: can they find the WC when they need to, for example? Can they move freely between the bedroom and the sitting area? If a demented person can find his or her way around a residential home, this can be regarded as successful coping behaviour. Primarily, the resident will be coping with the complexity of the home design, as he or she experiences it.

Residents' experience of the complexity of the home will depend primarily on overall design. This effect will be dominated by the design of those parts of the home that the residents actually use. Given this, it would be expected that the lay-out of group-living home designs, although more complex overall, would allow residents to restrict their use of the home to manageable limits. Thus one of the hypotheses tested was whether residents would find it easier to navigate their way around homes designed for group living.

The design of homes may also influence resident behaviour through the perceived 'normality' of the living arrangements. Normalisation theory (Wolfensberger, 1972) proposes that much of the behaviour of people in institutional settings is in response to a set of non-normal expectations which are reinforced by the architectural settings. Purpose-built institutions often do not fit in with the surrounding neighbourhood in design or scale. Internally these institutions are unlike domestic housing arrangements where most residents would previously have lived. Thus expectations of where things are likely to be (the bedrooms upstairs, for example) are constantly thwarted, leading to further confusion in demented residents trying to find their way around a strange building. There was no attempt in this study reported to incorporate a measure of 'normality' into the assessment of the physical environment as it was considered that none of the homes provided a sufficiently 'normal' environment for it to be possible to evaluate the effect on residents.

Assessing the home design

In order to make an assessment of the complexity of the buildings Lipman's (c.1983) schematic route diagram concept was employed. Lipman defines this as representing:

> the links between functional areas in a building when considered from the perspective of specific users who navigate themselves between such areas (Lipman, c.1983, p.2).

Those areas not normally used by the residents are excluded from the schematic diagram representing the home. The route diagram for staff members of a home would, therefore, be quite different to that for residents. From an architectural point of view these diagrams are a representation of the complexity of the circulation lay-outs of the homes.

The functional areas for the residents of a home for the elderly are bedroom areas, sitting areas, dining areas and WCs. The route diagram for a home consists of paths linking each of these zones and identifying the points where decisions have to be made. A decision point occurs whenever a zone is encountered or there is a junction of corridors. These can be simple (A), that is two-way decisions such that it is possible only to stay or to continue, or elaborate (B), usually three-way decisions.

Lipman (c.1983) conducted a study of eight homes in which the schematic route diagram for each was specified. These were ranked on a subjective assessment of their complexity made by a number of independent observers. From this, two measures of complexity were specified, one based on zones and the other on the number of decision points per resident weighted for complexity of decision. These measures were:

- the total number of zones in the home (including corridors)
- (A + 2B)/number of residents.

This implies that the more dispersed homes designed for group living are more complex and thus possibly unsuitable for the confused resident.

The approach was adapted for use in the study reported here by individualising the routes and incorporating some of the reservations that Lipman himself had expressed about the system. There were two main amendments:

- The diagrams used were specific to an individual and the use he or she made of the home. If residents in a group home never left their group area then that was all that was included on their route diagram.
- In addition to Lipman's decisions, exits from the route were included. A wrong decision at such a point would mean the resident being out of their usual section of the home or out of the building itself and thus more likely to become lost.

The route diagram for a resident in bedroom b1, in the example of a group home is shown in Figure 5.3. Although the overall lay-out of the home is complex, the route diagram is relatively straightforward because the resident in the normal course of events does not leave his or her group. The definition of 'in the normal course of events' for the study excluded those parts of the home the resident did not go to during a typical month.

For a resident in bedroom b1 in the example of a communal home, the route diagram is shown in Figure 5.4. The resident has to get to the one dining area in the home from an upstairs bedroom, so the route is necessarily long and has more decision points compared with that of the group home resident.

Each route diagram was scored and using these and the floor plans it was possible to ascertain the length of the route, average number of doors per corridor on the route, number of complex (B) and simple (A) decision points encountered and number of exits from the route. The total number of zones in the home as a whole was also recorded. These are shown on Figures 5.1 and 5.2. Corridors and sitting areas count individually as zones. Blocks of bedrooms separated by other facilities are counted as bedroom zones.

Distinctiveness and orientation aids

While residents' ability to find their way around has been represented as a 'coping response' to the design of the home, it is possible that it will also be affected by other environmental influences, such as the level of lighting. It might also be expected that residents would use 'landmarks' to help them find their way around. If so, orientation aids, such as colour-coding, might help residents find their way around. It would also be expected that many similar corridors would be more difficult to negotiate than a series of different

Figure 5.3
Route for residents in group home

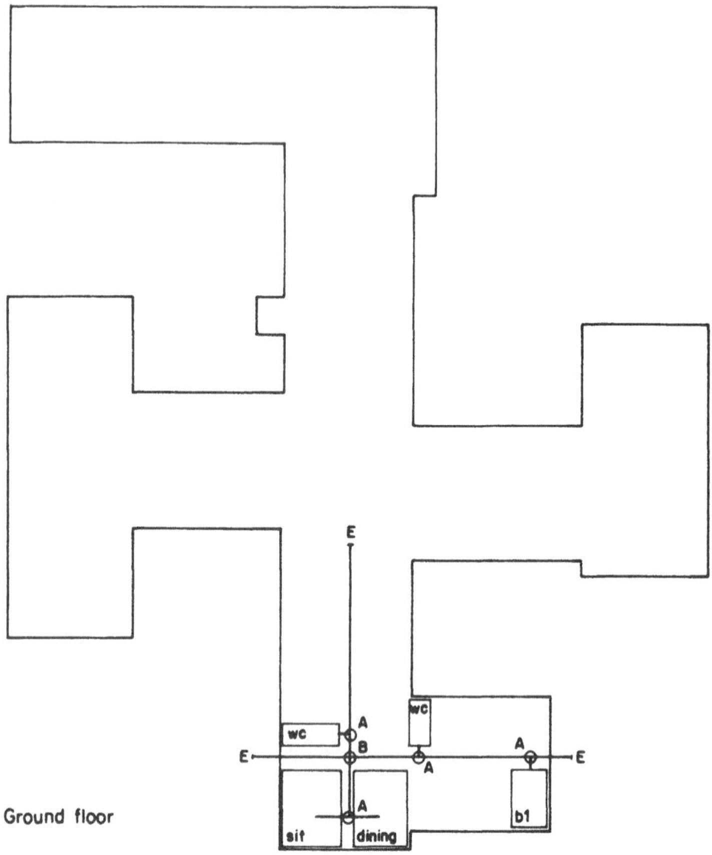

Route diagram score: simple A decisions 4; complex B decisions 1; exits from route 3; average doors per corridor 8. Route length 25 m.

spaces with distinctive aspects.

In addition to the routes and zones, therefore, a note was kept of the use in the home as a whole of colour-coding and large signs to indicate bedrooms and WCs. An attempt was made to assess the distinctiveness, both of aspects of the facility overall, and of sample residents' bedrooms and bedroom door. In practice, distinctiveness of various parts of the home proved an elusive concept to rate consistently as the halo effect of the overall attractiveness of

Figure 5.4
Route for residents in communal home

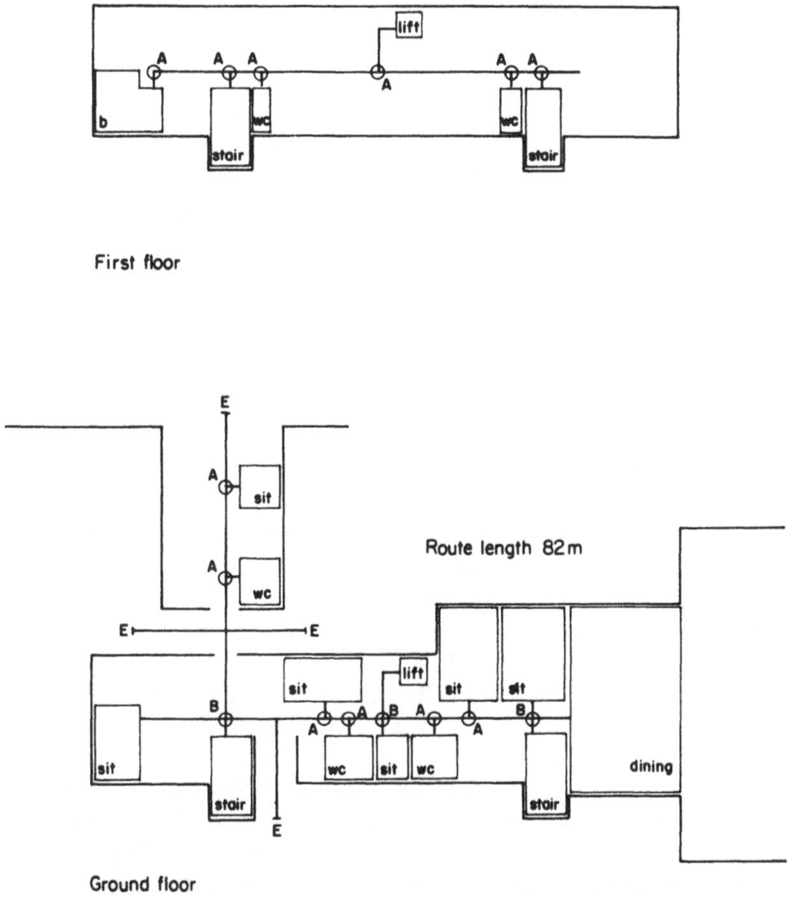

Route diagram score: simple A decisions 12; complex B decisions 3; exits from route 3; average doors per corridor 17. Route length 82 m.

the home tended to dominate ratings.

The use of colour-coding as an orientation aid appeared at times to be of dubious benefit. For example, in one specialist home brightly-coloured rugs and bedspreads were used as a method of colour-coding bedrooms. There appeared to be no attempt to assist the resident to use these as aids and the overall effect was of a home with virtually identical bedrooms. This was because the scope for personalisation of the bedrooms was even further restricted than in homes for elderly people generally. In other homes the use of colour-coding was often restricted by regulations or practice among those responsible for the decor at the local authority level. Generally, the main type of orientation aid used was clear labelling of doors, particularly WCs. In six of the homes the doors to WCs were clearly defined by colour, labelling or both. In only one home, however, were lounge areas defined clearly in this way.

Individual bedroom doors, and bedrooms upon entry, were rated by directly comparing them with neighbouring rooms. The question to be addressed was, simply, could this room or door be easily confused with those around, rather than the global assessment of distinctiveness of design. The majority (76 per cent) of bedroom doors had little to distinguish them from surrounding doors. In 27 per cent of cases the bedroom was clearly different on entry, but for 12 per cent of the sample the room appeared virtually identical to other bedrooms in the home. Although the remaining residents had rooms that could not be classified as identical, they were not distinct and could be confused with other bedrooms.

Assessing residents' ability to find their way around

The coping responses hypothesised in the model (see Chapter 2) can be represented as intermediate outcomes. These are outcomes which are often the expressed aim of an intervention, the link with such final outcomes as welfare being assumed. One such intermediate outcome is the level of engagement which has been used as an outcome measure in a number of studies (Jenkins et al., 1977; Rothwell et al., 1983). High engagement is often assumed to be linked with a high quality of life in such studies, although there is some debate about this assumption (Woods and Britton, 1985). In assessing the physical environment, an important intermediate outcome for demented residents is taken to be an ability to navigate themselves independently around the home and find the places where they wish to go. Inability to navigate the home successfully is hypothesised to affect adversely the welfare of residents by enforcing dependence on others.

A major difficulty is determining a useful measure of coping responses to the design of the home. If asked, residents may frequently not even know that they are in a home for elderly people. In practice, however, the same residents may be able to find their way to their bedrooms without difficulty. Observation of behaviour can lead to erroneous conclusions over a short period: is a person lost, wandering or simply taking the long way round?

A measure was devised by which it was hoped to overcome some of these difficulties. Staff who are dealing with residents on a daily basis know whether individuals can be relied on to find their own way to the WC, need reminding or are always taken by staff. As part of a questionnaire relating to each resident therefore, the officer-in-charge or a senior staff member was asked if that resident could find his or her way unaided (scoring 2), needed some directing (scoring 1) or had to be taken the whole way (scoring 0) between a few key places in the home:

- from the resident's usual sitting area to his or her bedroom,
- from the resident's usual sitting area to the dining area,
- from the resident's usual sitting area to the WC, and
- from the resident's bedroom to the WC.

The scores were added to provide a measure ('Find') that ranged from 8 to 0, the higher the score the better able a resident could find their way around.

Effects of home design on residents

Three main types of influence are likely to affect confused elderly residents' ability to find their way around a residential home:

- *personal*: degree of intellectual impairment, drugs taken and so on;
- *social*: features such as type of regime; and
- *physical*: lay-out of the home, for example.

The assumption in the model is that there will be interaction between the physical and social environment and the characteristics of the residents. To identify cause and effect, however hesitantly, necessitates breaking into this circuit and making assumptions about the rest of the influences. The interest here is to look at the effect of the physical environment given the dependency characteristics of individuals. If social effects are included in this kind of analysis, they can in some cases exclude the very effects with which the analysis is concerned.

For example, although in communal homes independence and self-disclosure were not related to residents' ability to move around the home, the levels of cohesion and conflict as measured by the SCES scales are related to the average number of doors per corridor (the correlation coefficients are -.61 and -.50 respectively). These latter dimensions of regime were also related to the number of exits on a route. More exits on a route are associated with higher cohesion (r=.59) and less conflict (r=-.41).

The levels of cohesion and conflict in a home could well be affected by the lay-out of a home: perhaps homes with long corridors tend to generate climates with a higher level of social distance and thus lower cohesion and conflict. Alternatively, residents' use of homes could be affected by the levels of cohesion and conflict in the social environment: perhaps those homes where there is a higher level of cohesion and lower conflict promote a feeling of confidence in residents such that they feel able to use more of the home and thus have more complex routes with more exits.

While the analysis of the relationship between the social environment and the ability of residents to find their way around is of interest, including social effects can exclude the physical characteristics of the environment, which is the focus of interest here. In the analysis described in this chapter, therefore, social effects have been excluded.

Regression analysis was used to analyse the relationship between the physical environment and the residents' ability to find their way around. Initially the residents CAPE Information/Orientation score was entered into the equation to reflect the fact that, for demented residents, degree of dementia, reflected by their general level of orientation, is a fundamental influence on spatial orientation in the home. Variables measuring personal and home design characteristics were then allowed to enter the equation using stepwise regression procedure. Aids to orientation were entered into the equation subsequently to examine whether they affected the impact of the home design on residents.

The initial analysis considered all the cases together. When the sample as a whole was analysed, the level of orientation accounted for 20 per cent of the variation in the Find measure. Orientation, mental ability, physical disability, number of zones, complex decisions, exits from the route and level of light in the home accounted for 51 per cent of the variation.

Although the variable indicating whether or not the home was based on a group design was not included in the equation, the signs of the coefficients led one to suppose that this might be an important factor. Positive coefficients for zones suggested that there might be a correlation between a higher number of zones and enhanced spatial orientation abilities among confused residents. This could be an indication that the more dispersed design of group homes was proving a positive influence in the management of confused elderly people. It was decided, therefore, to analyse the residents in group homes and communal homes separately to see if a clearer pattern emerged.

When the 51 residents of group homes were analysed as above, it was found that 25 per cent of the variation in residents' capacities to find their way around was explained by his or her level of orientation. For the 53 residents of the homes designed for communal living, only 15 per cent of the variation was explained. In other words, residents living in a group home would experience their level of orientation as a more important factor in finding their way around than residents living in a communal home. The reason for this becomes clearer when the variables in the different equations resulting from the separate analyses are examined. These are shown in Tables 5.2 and 5.3.

Communal homes

The personal characteristic that dominates the ability of residents to navigate communal homes successfully is their level of physical ability. This aspect of the residents had a highly significant coefficient while orientation and mental ability levels did not appear to be significant. The Find measure was based on whether staff had to take someone to their destination. Clearly, if they need help with walking they have to be escorted there. This either results in

Table 5.2
Communal homes

Variable	Coefficient	t -value	Sig.
Orientation	0.1	0.5	ns
Physical disability	-0.7	-5.9	***
Drugs	-0.9	-2.8	***
Zones	0.4	3.2	***
Exits	-0.3	-3.2	***
A decisions	0.2	2.3	**
Doors per corridor	-0.1	-1.7	*
Constant	-7.2	-2.8	***

Dependent variable = 'Find': resident's ability to find his/her way around the home

$R^2 = .65$
Adjusted $R^2 = .60$
n = 53
ns not significant
* $p < .10$
** $p < .05$
*** $p < .01$

Table 5.3
Group-living homes

Variable	Coefficient	t -value	Sig.
Orientation	0.3	1.9	*
Mental ability	0.2	2.2	**
Physical disability	-0.4	-3.2	***
Light	2.1	3.3	***
B decisions	1.6	3.4	***
Length of route	-0.02	-2.4	**
Doors per corridor	0.3	1.8	*
Constant	-6.3	-1.5	ns

Dependent variable = 'Find': resident's ability to find his/her way around the home

$R^2 = 0.65$
Adjusted $R^2 = 0.59$
n = 51
ns not significant
* $p < .1$
** $p < .05$
*** $p < .01$

the staff perceiving them as unable to find their way or, because they never have to think about where they are going, actual inability to find their way. In either case the resident becomes undesirably dependent on staff.

In homes designed for communal living, the more psychotropic drugs a resident received the less likely he or she was to be able to find their way around. This is not reflected in the group homes. It is possible that this is because more of the group homes are specialist and would have, perhaps, more in-house expert knowledge and better links with the psychogeriatric services (Arie and Jolley, 1982). Such drugs could thus be expected to be more appropriately prescribed and administered.

The design characteristics that appeared to assist residents most were simple decision points and a larger number of zones in the home as a whole. These characteristics were associated with homes that were converted from older establishments.

The more doors there were in a corridor on average (a feature that generally indicated longer corridors) the more confusing the communal home for its residents. If measures of social environment were allowed to enter the equation, a higher level of conflict in communal homes appears to result in an increase in the ability of residents to avoid getting lost. A more likely interpretation is that the long corridors adversely affect a resident's navigational skills, and this kind of lay-out (shown in Figure 5.2) affects the social climate of the home.

In the communal homes the more exit points on the route, the more likely a resident was to get lost. However, this does not apply in group-living homes and may reflect the fact that the greater flexibility of designs for group-living enables residents to set their own boundaries. Having made the judgement themselves, they may be more likely to remember it, or repeat it. In communal homes the central dining area may mean residents are forced into areas of the home that they find confusing.

Group-living homes

In group-living homes both mental and physical personal characteristics of residents are important influences on their ability to find their way. Physical disability is an important variable, but as the distances between the zones are so much less than in communal homes, fewer residents are likely to be assisted by staff for physical reasons. Thus orientation and mental ability remain significant factors in group-living homes.

As in communal homes an important design characteristic was the number of decision points. These appeared to assist residents in moving from one area to another. In group-living homes, however, it was the more complex decisions that were significant. The contrast with communal homes was also reflected in the direction of influence of the average number of doors per corridor. In group-living homes residents were better able to cope with more doors per corridor.

One interesting relationship is the importance of the lighting level in group-living homes. It is not surprising that additional light has a positive effect on residents' abilities. The level of light tended to be lower in the homes designed for group living than in communal homes, possibly due to the frequency of internal corridors heavily dependent on artificial lighting. Staff might simply be forgetting to switch lights on. Defunct bulbs that have not been replaced may also make such areas very dark, even in the middle of the day. Either could create unnecessary confusion for the residents.

Residents who had longer routes in the group homes experienced more difficulty. This probably reflects the effect of residents who wander. Such residents will roam the whole building with little idea of where they are at all, let alone in which part of the home.

Discussion

One question that inevitably arises in a discussion of the physical environment of homes for demented elderly people is what type of design is most favourable. Two particular issues have emerged from the analysis of complexity of design and its effect on residents: the contrast between the effects of designs for communal or group living, and a concept that gives coherence to the apparently contradictory results: meaningful decisions.

The separate analysis of the effects of group and communal homes makes the task of directly contrasting the two types of design difficult. In order to facilitate comparison, an equation was estimated in which the only environmental factor included was a dummy variable for group-living designs. Although the coefficient was not statistically significant, this might be because of the greater degree of impairment of residents in the specialist homes which were predominantly designed for group living. The CAPE measure of orientation included to adjust for this could be insufficiently sensitive in this context.

The issue is not clear cut, but there would appear to be a case in favour of the current trend towards group-living designs:

- The level of control residents have over their routes is enhanced in group designs as shown by the reduced influence of physical disability and the negative impact of the exits from the routes in communal homes.
- The homes were ranked by estimating the average predicted Find score (using the equations in Tables 5.2 and 5.3) for residents if physical and mental disability were held constant. This resulted in all the group-living homes predicting a higher average Find measure than the communal homes. Moreover, the two homes that had been converted from private housing appeared the least confusing of all the communal homes. That is, those least like the traditional communal design appear to have the most favourable effect. The best group home on this basis is shown in Figure

5.1 and the worst communal design in Figure 5.2.

One question that arises from the above analysis concerns the dependence of directions of influence on the overall type of design. Why is it that longer corridors are an aid in group designs and a disadvantage in communal designs? Why are simple decisions important in communal homes and complex decisions important in group homes? Is there a common theme that can link these apparently disparate results?

One possible link is the concept of meaningful decisions or landmarks. In a communal home, such as that shown in Figure 5.2, simple decisions tend to occur when a sitting area or other zone is encountered. Places that are actually used by residents are likely to mean something to them: at such a point they have to think about where they are going. If a corridor is too long they may forget where they are going by the time the next decision point is reached.

The positive effect of elaborate decisions in group homes also supports this concept of using the decision points as landmarks. Given the usual design features of homes for the elderly, these elaborate decisions tend to occur where bedrooms or doors to communal areas are positioned on junctions, or when dining and seating facilities are in the same area. Again these are places that are used very frequently, and are therefore more memorable to the residents.

Using this framework an unhelpful design would result when there were a lot of meaningless decisions. In communal homes this would occur when there were few identifiable zones and long corridors with lots of doors. In group homes this might occur when there were many short corridors within the group sections, forming a maze effect. Figure 5.5 illustrates a single group home where there are a number of corridor junctions, few of which are likely to have any particular meaning to the residents.

Thus meaningful decisions as landmarks would anticipate the results achieved: a negative effect from doors per corridor in communal homes, a positive effect in group homes. Simple decisions in communal homes provide aids where there are long corridors. In group homes the more complex decisions are more distinctive. Although there was little evidence of effectiveness of orientation aids used in the homes, there is clearly a role for such aids in reinforcing messages to residents. This analysis suggests that orientation aids would be most effective when used in conjunction with meaningful decision points for residents.

Conclusion

The aspect of the physical environment investigated in most detail was the relationship between design complexity and residents' ability to find their way around. The analysis was essentially exploratory in approach so the

Figure 5.5
The 'maze' effect in a group home

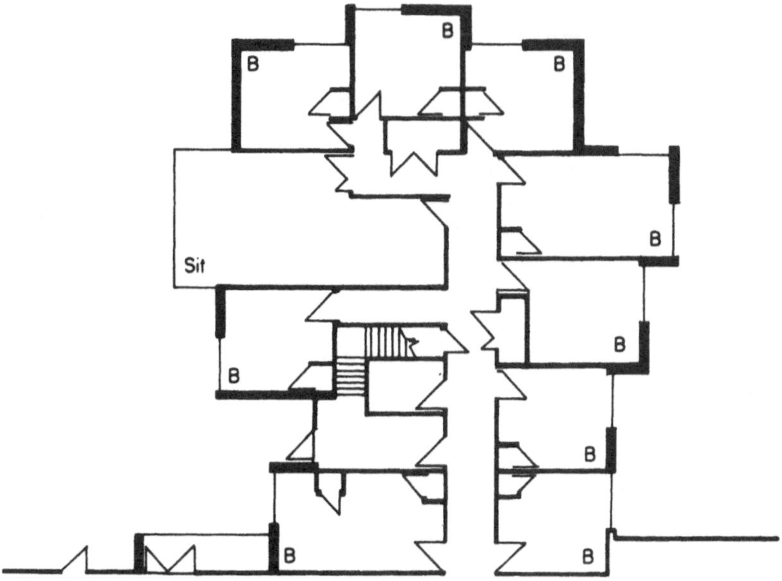

conclusions drawn should be treated with some care. The coping response measure (residents' ability to find their way around a home) was newly devised and therefore not authenticated. The inclusion of observation techniques or asking residents themselves the way to various locations in the home would have provided a check on the validity of the measure and should ideally be incorporated in any future work. Moreover, although the thirteen homes provided a good variety of design features, they were not comprehensive in covering all types of design.

However, with those reservations in mind, the analysis provides a useful starting point for further work. The Find measure, if validated, could prove a useful tool for assessing the impact of the physical environment on demented elderly people. Individual route diagrams may also form the basis of an approach to providing a picture of residents' experiences of their environment and demonstrate how their use of a building is influenced both by the design and their competence.

For those concerned with designing facilities, the results would support the current trend towards group living in homes for elderly people. Designs which enable people to restrict their use of a building to, for example, one or two short corridors and associated rooms will enhance the independence of both physically and cognitively-impaired people. The results do suggest, though, that adequate lighting is key in such designs for people with confusional difficulties. Moreover, design features which reinforce the purpose of decision points in a normalistic way – such as a clear view of dining facilities in a dining area – should serve to enhance natural landmarks. Group homes will allow those who need more physical activity room to wander and/or take exercise. Moreover, the results in Chapter 3 suggest that enclosed grounds in which it is clearly safe to wander may encourage staff to facilitate residents' use of outdoor areas.

In the examination of the concept of personal territory there was some evidence to support the hypothesis that the 'own chair' culture is a response by the home to limited personal territory for residents. The concepts are elusive to measure, however, and no firm conclusions can be drawn. The need now is to turn to an examination of the impact of these environmental influences, both direct and indirect, on the behaviour and orientation of residents.

6 The effect of the environment of residential homes on demented residents

Certain aspects of care, such as maintaining dignity and respect for privacy, are generally regarded as desirable attributes of residential care *per se*. Other issues, such as the importance of activities and types of regime that are suitable for elderly people with confusional difficulties, are open to debate. Ultimately, decisions about these should depend upon the effect on residents: the outcomes of care. The purpose of this chapter is to estimate a model which relates aspects of the supra-personal, social and physical environment described in previous chapters to outcomes for the sample residents, providing a contribution to these more debatable issues.

Methodology

To recap, the social ecological model introduced in Chapter 2 is one in which changes in competence and behaviour are a function of personal and environmental influences. This is not a straightforward relationship and, for the purpose of exploring the data to identify environmental effects, simplification of the underlying model is required. For example, coping responses are hypothesised to intervene between many aspects of the environment and behavioural change. Where these cannot be measured directly they can be represented by the relationship between specified environmental variables and the measures of outcome.

Regression analysis was used to estimate a four-equation model of environmental effect. Table 6.1 lists all the variables included in the exploratory analysis. The four dependent variables were all indicators of outcomes for residents at the end of the six-month study period. Some of the problems in measuring outcomes were discussed in Chapter 2. While the ultimate outcome or final output of a service is the welfare of the client or resident, a reliable measure of welfare for demented people has yet to be identified and the approach here was to define outcomes in terms of behaviour and orientation. Changes in the CAPE scales of apathy, social disturbance, and information/orientation formed three of the outcome measures. An indicator of contentedness as judged by staff which recorded the level of smiling and agitation displayed by residents formed the basis of the fourth outcome measure. The

Table 6.1
Variables included in the analysis

Variable	Description	Observed range
Outcome		
Change in apathy	High score = increased apathy (CAPE Ap)	-6 to +5
Change in social disturbance	High score = increased soc. disturb. (CAPE Sd)	-4 to +4
Change in orientation	High score = increased orientation (CAPE I/O)	-4 to +5
Change in discontentedness	High score = more agitated, less smiling	-2 to +2
Personal characteristics		
Length of stay	Number of years in the home	0.5 to 10
Initial levels of:		
Depression	2= no symptoms of depression	2 to 8
Apathy	0= low apathy	0 to 10
Social disturbance	0= low social disturbance	0 to 9
Orientation	0= low orientation	0 to 9
Discontentedness	0= low agitation, high smiling	0 to 4
Mental ability, time 1	0= low mental ability (CAPE MAb score)	0 to 11
Change in mental ability	High score = increased mental ability	-8 to +7
Physical disability, time 1	0= no disabilities (CAPE Pd)	1 to 12
Communication difficulties	0= no difficulties (CAPE Cd)	0 to 4
Hearing difficulties	0= can hear without aids	0,1
Age	Age in years	68 to 97
Gender	1 = male 2 = female	1,2
Environmental influences		
Psychotropic drugs	Number of different drugs taken	0 to 6
Supra-personal		
Specialist	1= home designated specialist	0,1
Day care	1= day care clients in the home	0,1
Short-stay	% of short-stay residents	0 to 7.7
Confused residents	% of residents moderately/severely confused	5.1 to 100
Resident turnover	no. of residents left/number of residents in home (Chapter 3)	0.4 to 1.4
Staff turnover	% of staff left during six-month study period	0 to 20
Staff sickness	Average days sick per staff member	0.6 to 5.3
Care staff-resident ratio	Number of care staff per resident	0.2 to 0.4
Social work staff	% of staff with social work qualification	0 to 20
Nursing staff	% of staff with nursing qualification	0 to 30
Trained staff	% of staff with in-service training	6 to 57
Qualified staff	% of staff with any qualification	7 to 79

Table 6.1 (continued)
Variables included in the analysis

Variable	Description	Observed range
Social		
SCES subscales: cohesion, conflict, independence, self-disclosure, organisation, resident influence, physical comfort (see Chapter 4 for description)		
Restrictive regime	1= home has restrictive regime (see Chapter 4)	0,1
Positive regime	1= home has positive regime (see Chapter 4)	0,1
Activities	No. of activity sessions per month	0.7 to 48
Engagement in activities	Individual resident's monthly rate of activities	0 to 55
Frequency of visitors	Number of visits per month	0 to 30
Friends (staff/resident)	1= has special friend(s) among staff or residents	0,1
Bedtime set by staff	1= bedtime set by staff	0,1
Formal care plan/policy	1= resident has care plan/policy	0,1
Access to grounds	1= resident may use grounds unaccompanied	0,1
Private place	1= has place can lock small items	0,1
Chooses what to wear	1= chooses daily clothing	0,1
Personalisation of bedroom	1= room clearly personalised	0,1
Physical		
Light	High score= bright	3 to 9
Quiet	High score= quiet	6 to 10
Most residents have 'own' chair	1= > 75% of residents sit in particular chair	0,1
Single room	1= has single bedroom	0,1
Bedroom space	Square metres of bedroom area	2 to 11
Change of bedroom	1= changed room in six-month period of study	0,1
Find way around the home	Ability to find way around (see Chapter 5)	0 to 8

scoring of this variable was such that an increased score reflected less smiling and more agitation and has thus been termed 'discontentedness' here.

For each outcome an equation was estimated. The level of each dependent variable (social disturbance, apathy, orientation and discontentedness) at the beginning of the study period was included to control for the initial state of the sample resident. The initial level of apathy, for example, is a fundamental influence on the degree to which apathy is likely to increase. An indicator of depression (see Chapter 2) was also included to allow, in the absence of clinical diagnosis, for the degree to which any effects were due to depressive rather than organic causes. Third, the length of stay of the individual in the institution indicated for how long they had been exposed to the present environment or treatment.

The remaining variables reflecting personal characteristics (see Table 6.1) were then included in the equations using stepwise analysis. This set of variables reflected abilities or competence and descriptive factors such as gender. It was hypothesised that these each might affect the underlying rate of deterioration or pattern of the disease so any effects needed to be allowed for before investigating the impact of the variables of real interest: those reflecting different aspects of the environment.

Once the personal characteristics associated with changes in each outcome measure had been included in each equation, the environmental variables were included. The only purely personal environmental effect included was the number of psychotropic drugs being taken. These are sometimes used to control abnormal behaviours and inappropriate usage has been shown in some residential homes (Wade et al., 1986). Ideally the expected effect of each drug should be incorporated in the model. A simpler measure of the number of psychotropic drugs taken can, however, provide an indicator of use and likelihood of adverse reactions.

The indicators of the supra-personal environment reflected the functions of the home and the characteristics of staff and residents. For the social and physical dimensions, indicators were included of both the overall environment (level of light and type of regime, for example) and individual experience (size of bedroom space and whether the resident is allowed to choose clothes each day, for example) of that environment. Only one coping response was included: residents' ability to find their way around the homes. Both the individual experience and the coping response reflected an interaction between individual competence and environmental impact hypothesised in the model.

After the equations had been estimated and examined for consistency on theoretical grounds, they were estimated as a structural equation model using LISREL (Jöreskog and Sörbom, 1986). There are two principal reasons why the relationship between changes in behaviour and orientation in demented residents should be represented as a structural equation model in which a set of equations are estimated simultaneously.

- Each outcome measure refers to a change in the same individual. It might well be that someone who reacts to a negative environmental influence with apathy is less likely to exhibit socially-disturbed behaviour. Thus, changes in apathy and socially-disturbed behaviour would be expected to co-vary although no causal connection would be implied. Even if common causes of changes in behaviour had not been identified, it would be reasonable to suppose that the underlying progressive nature of the condition might affect each of the outcome measures. This again implies a covariance between the outcome measures.

- By estimating each equation separately there is a risk of excluding the influence of the other equations and thus mis-specifying the model. There is also inefficiency in that not all the available information has been used in the estimation procedure.

Table 6.2 shows the estimated coefficients of the standardised model using LISREL. In the following discussion the impact of personal characteristics and each aspect of the environment (personal, supra-personal, social and physical) is discussed in turn.

Personal characteristics

The high level of significance and negative effect of the initial level of each outcome measure on changes in each measure reflects the limited nature of the scales. Once a high level of problematic behaviour or very low level of orientation is indicated, there is a limit to the amount deterioration can be measured. This is important to note because it suggests that the results of the model may have limited applicability to very severely demented people as changes in orientation and/or behaviour over the six months may not have been recorded.

Of the two variables included to allow for the research design (depression and length of stay), length of stay did not have a significant effect on the behavioural outcomes, but a longer period in the home was associated with less deterioration in orientation. This may indicate the benefit of a better knowledge of the environment, perhaps among those residents whose cognitive abilities have deteriorated while living in the home. The existence of depressive symptoms at the beginning of the study period, on the other hand, was associated with behavioural outcomes. The more depressed a resident was at the beginning of the study period, the higher the chance of there being a deterioration in socially-disturbed behaviour and a deterioration in contentedness: the level of smiling was likely to decrease and/or agitation increase. Neither apathy nor orientation was affected, however.

The apparent effect of communication difficulties in reducing socially-disturbed behaviour that was found may reflect a tendency among people with communication difficulties to withdraw rather than express their frustration. Certainly the initial level of apathy was more closely associated with communication difficulties (r=.39) than social disturbance (r=.01).

The results suggest that the better oriented residents are, the more apathetic they are likely to become. Again this may be the effect of a restricted scale. The very regressed who score zero on the orientation scale will have little ability to engage, and will thus appear very apathetic. This interpretation is supported by a negative relationship between apathy and orientation at the beginning of the study period (r=-.34). The orientation of residents who had

Table 6.2
Estimated model of environmental effect

DEPENDENT VARIABLE

	Change in social disturbance	Change in apathy	Change in orientation	Change in discontented-ness
Personal characteristics				
Depression	0.18 *	-0.03 ns	-0.05 ns	0.34 ***
Length of stay	0.09 ns	0.07 ns	0.18 *	0.01 ns
Social disturbance	-0.57 ***	–	–	–
Apathy	–	-0.65 ***	–	–
Orientation	–	-0.22 *	-0.65 ***	–
Contentedness	–	–	–	-0.76 ***
Communication difficulties	-0.25 **	–	–	–
Mental ability	–	–	0.61 ***	–
Environment characteristics				
Psychotropic drugs	0.22 **	0.18 *	–	–
Turnover of residents	0.25 *	–	–	–
Staff sickness	–	0.21 **	–	–
Care staff-resident ratio	–	-0.24 **	–	–
Nursing staff	–	0.26 ***	0.49 ***	–
Staff turnover	–	–	-0.54 ***	–
Positive regime	-0.22 **	-0.22 **	0.22 *	–
Frequency of visitors	–	–	0.23 **	–
Chooses what to wear	-0.16 *	–	–	–
Quiet	-0.36 ***	–	0.47 ***	–
Find	–	-0.32 ***	–	-0.26 ***
Most residents have 'own' chair	–	–	–	0.32 ***
R^2	.53	.44	.46	.52
number of residents = 78				

Total coefficient of determination = 0.949
Chi-square with 47 df = 37.05 (p=.851)
Goodness of Fit Index = 0.965
Adjusted Goodness of Fit Index = 0.774

ns p > .10
* p < .10
** p < .05
** p < .01

a higher level of mental ability at the beginning of the study period was less likely to deteriorate over the six-month period.

Psychotropic drugs

Only one aspect of the personal system was included as part of the environmental influences because, as a direct treatment, it may be influenced by the policy of the home. This was the number of psychotropic drugs a resident was taking at the beginning of the study period. Additional drugs may be prescribed in an attempt to control deteriorating behaviour. The higher the number of drugs taken, however, the more likely the incidence of adverse reactions or difficult behaviour (Wade et al., 1986). This study also found an association between the number of different psychotropic drugs being taken and increased socially-disturbed behaviour and apathy, suggesting that drugs were being inappropriately prescribed and/or administered in the homes.

Supra-personal environmental influences

Only one of the indicators reflecting the characteristics of the resident population of the homes was associated with any of the measures of outcome. Turnover of residents was related to increased social disturbance of the sample residents. Turnover was measured by the number who left the home during the period divided by the number of residents in the homes at the beginning of the study. This was 91 per cent on average. Only 21 per cent of people entering the homes during the period were new admissions, however, and only 11 per cent of the residents died. The high resident turnover figure reflected the combined effects of holidays, short-term hospitalisation and short-term care. The proportion of residents who had been admitted on a short-term basis was very small but was still double the national average of 2 per cent. This was because the majority of the homes (eight) were located in one authority in which over 4 per cent of residents were in the homes on a short-stay basis. In the three other authorities less than 1 per cent of residents were short-stay.

It is probable that a higher turnover may be associated with a less settled and predictable atmosphere. Even in group-living homes residents will be living with many more people than they did before admission and such changes in atmosphere could conceivably compound the difficulty of adjusting to a communal lifestyle. Or simply the change in the faces and different social atmosphere resulting from different people may be sufficient to have a deleterious effect on behaviour.

The dominating supra-personal influence, however, was the staffing of the homes. Staff to resident ratio, turnover and sickness among staff, and the numbers of staff with nursing qualifications are all associated with resident outcomes.

Willcocks et al. (1987) found that homes with a higher number of staff-resident hours and more part-time staff were more likely to have resident-oriented practices, but Lemke and Moos (1986) found that staffing levels were unrelated to indicators of quality of care. Bond et al. (1989) suggest that there may be a level of staffing at which an increase in staff makes no difference to quality of care but below which care suffers. If this is so the results here would suggest that the level of staffing in the study was below this threshold. In the study homes the average number of hours of staff time per working week per resident, for all grades of staff, was 21; the same as the number of hours of staff time per resident nationally in 1981 (Darton and Wright, 1989). This staff-resident ratio results in an average of twelve hours of care staff time per resident.

The results also suggest that a low turnover of staff has a positive influence on residents. Staff turnover in the study homes was not unduly high on average, although given the reliance on part-time staff in residential care of elderly people (68 per cent of the staff in the study homes worked part-time) it would not be surprising if turnover of staff was high. In one home 19 per cent of these members of staff left during the six-month period. However, on average only 7 per cent of these grades of staff left, and 72 per cent of the 244 care and supervisory staff who completed questionnaires had been in post for over two years.

This result corresponds with other findings. A high turnover of staff has been found to be related to lower levels of physical care of nursing home residents in the USA (Garibaldi et al., 1981). Moreover, Stryker (1981) suggests that depression, disengagement, disorientation and isolation will increase when relationships between staff and residents are disrupted by changes among staff members. Indeed the result provides a parallel with another finding in the study: the effect of turnover among other residents on the sample residents. It is probable that familiar faces provide a useful reminder and aid to orientation and that longer-established staff will be more familiar with residents and their personal histories. If staff can understand residents' individual backgrounds they may link in better to conversations and positively reinforce fact rather than fiction (Feil, 1985).

However stable the staff population and whatever the ratio of staff to residents on paper, consistency and contact levels in practice can be low if there is a high level of sickness among staff. Time taken off by staff as a result of sickness was related to changes in residents' levels of apathy. During the six-month study period, care and supervisory staff had two days sick leave each on average. This ranged from an average of five days per staff member in one home to about half a day in another. The six-month period of the study was during the winter, a time of the year when sickness levels would be expected to be relatively high. Discussion with officers-in-charge established that the overall level of sickness among staff did not appear to present a problem on a routine basis. Management difficulties arose when an outbreak of influenza resulted in a lot of staff being away from work at one time, or chronic illness resulted in long-term understaffing. The evidence here would suggest that these periods directly affect residents.

Sickness, staff turnover and staff to resident ratio are indicators of the level of availability of staff to residents which in turn will affect whether there is the opportunity to stimulate and motivate those residents most prone to becoming apathetic. It is interesting to note also that the rate of sickness among care staff showed a high negative correlation to the level of in-service training (r=-.67). It could be hypothesised that low motivation among staff could be reflected in a higher tendency to take days off when sick. Alternatively, poorly-motivated staff may experience higher stress, resulting in increased levels of sickness. If in-service training succeeds in increasing staff motivation, then a negative association between sickness and in-service training would be expected. Such an interpretation would suggest that even if the training itself does not feed directly through to benefit residents, any consequent reduction in the amount of sick leave taken by care staff may well do so.

The proportion of staff with nursing qualifications was directly associated with outcomes, however. Overall, 13 per cent of staff had nursing qualifications of some sort, a level close to the national average (Darton, 1983). One relationship is the opposite of that which might be expected: a higher proportion of staff with nursing qualifications is associated with an increased level of apathy. While not suggesting that staff with a background in general nursing will actively encourage apathy, this may reflect hospital ward experience. In general wards, apathy may simply not be experienced as a problem. Quiet patients can be seen in this context as 'good' and 'no trouble'. The concept that staff with general nursing backgrounds might not see apathy as a problem would again suggest that motivation among staff is an important influence on resident behaviour. However, in contrast to their apparent effect on apathy, nursing qualifications seem to have a beneficial influence on the orientation of residents. This may reflect a higher level of understanding of the condition or a more professional attitude to caring for people with senile dementia.

Social environmental influences

The hypothesis that the benefit of a low turnover among staff was in part due to continuity of contact would be supported by one of the effects of the social environment: a positive association between a high frequency of visitors and improved orientation. In addition to familiarity and continuity, visiting can be seen as an effective form of stimulation, in which residents are likely to be motivated to respond, and in which they get one-to-one attention.

One aspect of the social environment dominated the results, however: the association between the existence of a positive regime and improvements in three of the outcomes – social disturbance, apathy and orientation. As an experimental method of describing homes, this association between a positive regime and behaviour provides evidence in favour of the validity of the measure. While the description does not provide direct practice implications for the care of demented elderly people, it does provide a method of relating a set of influences on outcomes for confused residents. The homes with a positive regime encouraged the independence and influence of the residents more than the other homes. It would seem likely that those homes that actively encourage independence would encourage staff to seek out and be aware of residents becoming apathetic and withdrawn. The level of cohesion and organisation in these homes is also generally higher, providing a more supportive environment to those with orientation and behavioural difficulties.

The comprehensive nature of the association between positive regimes and favourable outcomes has important policy implications both for the measure itself and the need to identify key characteristics of the regimes and influences on their formation. This is explored further in Chapter 7.

The choice over what to wear each day was included as an individual indicator of the attitude to the resident. Where residents chose what they wore, it was hypothesised that they would tend to be encouraged to exert control over their daily lives. Various studies have emphasised the importance of locus of control in the welfare of elderly people generally (Palmore and Luikhert, 1972; Challis, 1981). It is probable that the same should apply to elderly people with dementia – perhaps being all the more important because capacity for control is so reduced in people with this condition. If the assumption is correct that choice over daily clothes reflects a level of control over daily life, the results suggest that lack of control over daily decision-making may be a factor in socially-disturbed behaviour.

Physical environmental influences

It was hypothesised that a quiet, settled atmosphere would have a positive effect on orientation (Feier and Leight, 1981) and this was found to be the case. A noisy atmosphere, particularly when the noise comes from a number of different sources, can be confusing. There may be a tendency for demented residents to shut out a noisy atmosphere. This may in turn lead to an increased sense of disorientation. The association with increased social disturbance suggests that a high noise level may also have a disruptive effect on residents. Residents 'setting one another off' was reported anecdotally during the study: if one resident starts shouting or moaning, other demented residents will frequently follow suit. In the previous chapter another major source of noise in homes was noted: television sets often had the volume set high to aid residents with hearing difficulties.

The effect of the physical complexity of the homes was hypothesised to act on resident behaviour via the 'coping response' of residents finding their way around. Coping responses, such as observed engagement, are often taken as measures of outcome (Felce and Jenkins, 1979; McCormack and Whitehead, 1981), the assumption being that a positive coping response is likely to be associated with an increase in welfare. Some support for this assumption was found in the case of spatial orientation, as an ability to navigate the home was found to be associated with a beneficial effect on apathy. This would suggest that if residents cannot find their way to where they want to go, after a while they may give up and become less inclined to try to initiate activity. The results of the analysis also suggest that residents who can navigate around the home are more contented, being less likely to become agitated and more likely to smile.

Although the 'own chair' culture is a social phenomenon, it is hypothesised to be an aspect of territoriality, resulting from lack of personal territory in the home as a whole (see Chapter 5). This was associated with increased agitation and reduced smiling among demented residents, suggesting that residents with a poorly-developed sense of ownership and territory find it difficult to cope in a home where such issues are dominant in the character or culture of the home. The outcome measure was intended to capture the type of outcomes important to staff on a day-to-day basis and has been interpreted as an indicator of contentedness. Homes where there is an emphasis on cultural norms and unwritten rules may provide a poor 'fit' for residents with dementia, resulting in a feeling of discontent, unrelieved by any possibility that such residents can do anything to change this aspect of their environment.

The possibility that the environmental effects on the indicator of contentedness were interdependent was explored on the basis that the index may primarily reflect residents' level of agitation. Residents who cannot find their way around the home may have additional difficulties in a social climate in which sitting in the wrong chair is actively discouraged. If a resident cannot find his or her chair and is not allowed to sit elsewhere, agitation may well ensue! An interaction term, indicating the level of ability of the resident only when he or she was in a home with this 'own chair' culture, did not prove to be statistically significant or add to the explanatory power of the equation, however, and the 'own chair' effect may merely reflect a more rigid attitude among residents, leading to frustration in demented residents.

Overall effect of the environment

The fundamental hypothesis of the investigation was that the residential care environment has an impact on residents' behaviour. One method of assessing the importance of the environmental effects as a whole is to examine the change in the explanatory power of the equation when environmental influences are included. For the model as a whole the inclusion of the environmental effects did result in a significant improvement in explanatory power, in so far as this can be judged using LISREL (Netten, 1990). It is of more interest, however, to look at the overall environmental effect on the individual measures of outcome.

A significant proportion of the variation in each outcome variable was attributable to environmental influences when the equations were estimated separately. For social disturbance the proportion of variation explained by environmental variables was quite low (R^2 increased by .15). This was sufficient, however, to reject the null hypothesis that the environment as a whole did not affect social disturbance. Although the proportion of variation in apathetic behaviour explained by environmental influences was not much higher (R^2 increased by .19), this was 40 per cent of the variation explained by the equation as a whole. An even higher proportion of the change in orientation was attributable to the environmental influences. The increase in R^2 was .24, more than doubling the proportion of variation explained. For discontentedness, however, the environmental variables only contributed a further .07 to the R^2, although again this was a significant increase suggesting that this devised measure is reflecting, if only to a limited degree, some of the demented residents' responses to environmental influences.

In evaluating the model it is also necessary to examine the assumptions made about those residents for whom outcome measures were not available: those who died or left the home during the study period. Analysis of the predicted outcomes of those who died or were temporarily in hospital confirmed that an assumption that these occurrences were random was reasonable. However, this assumption was not tenable for those who were permanently transferred whether to another residential home or to hospital. Indeed, analysis of residents who were permanently transferred showed that they had more behavioural difficulties at the start of the study and the model does not provide satisfactory predicted scores. Given the low number of residents who were 'lost' in this way (five) the source of bias in estimation is relatively limited. However, if, as suggested by the influence of the starting values of each outcome measure, other effects are contributing to this source of bias, then the model will not adequately predict the effect of the environment on more severely demented residents.

One home (Centrelea) proved of particular interest in this respect as two of the five residents who were transferred were in the home at the start of the study. Only four residents were included in the study from Centrelea and the two survivors had a higher level of social disturbance at the end of the study period than would have been predicted by the model. It is therefore of interest to see how the initial circumstances for the four residents differed from that of other residents in the sample and to see whether the clues to the 'omitted influences' conflict or concur with the interpretation of the results so far.

The values of all the variables included in the analysis (identified in Table 6.1) were examined to identify in what way, if any, characteristics of sample residents in this home and the home itself differed from the other residents and homes. Of the personal characteristics the only significant differences found were that the residents of Centrelea were more physically disabled and socially disturbed than in the other homes. The higher level of physical disability was interesting to note, especially in the context that the residents of this home were also significantly less able to find their way around. Wheelchairs were noticeably more in evidence in this home where corridors were long and the dining area distant from many of the sitting areas. There was no evidence that the sample residents of this home had more underlying mental problems than residents of other homes: their average score for mental ability was higher (5.8) compared to the other homes (4.5).

In the home as a whole there were fewer residents judged to be moderately or severely confused, which is what would be expected in a non-specialist home and no residents at the time of the initial approach to the home were short-stay. There was a lower level of conflict in Centrelea than in the other homes (using the SCES subscale) and there was a stable staffing situation with a low turnover and rate of sickness compared with the other study homes. These factors are unlikely to contribute to higher social disturbance. However, significantly fewer staff had social work qualifications and the SCES subscale of organisation was higher. All the sample residents had set bedtimes and none of these residents had personalised their rooms to any obvious degree, suggesting that the 'locus of control' was heavily biased towards the institution rather than the residents.

In comparing the residents on the basis of variables included in the model, none of the sample residents in the home was taking psychotropic drugs, and turnover of residents was close to the average of the other homes. The proportion of staff who had nursing qualifications was close to the average at 11 per cent and the staff-resident ratio was also about average. Staff turnover and sickness, on the other hand, were significantly lower than average. The social environment was reflected in a mixed regime in which none of the sample residents had choice over daily clothes but had a similar number of visitors to other sample residents. All of the indicators of the physical environment in the model were significantly 'worse' in this home: it was noisier, more territorial (residents had their 'own chair' in a communal area) and residents were significantly less likely to be able to find their way around.

The overall picture that emerges from these relationships is of a home which is run generally more to the benefit of the staff than the demented residents. It is easier to take someone in a wheelchair than to guide and reinforce routes. It is easier to choose for demented residents than assist them to choose. It is also easier to put residents to bed when it suits staff, if the residents cannot find their way and need assistance. There is no implication here that the staff do not intend to care well for the residents. The need to care for these residents, however, is expressed in a need to do things *for* residents and a tendency, perhaps, to underestimate their ability. The short-term results might be a more efficient use of time; the long-term results, however, are reflected in a higher level of social disturbance in demented residents.

Conclusion

The aim of the analysis was to establish important influences on outcomes for elderly people with confusional difficulties in residential care and was essentially exploratory in nature. The full list of variables included in the analysis is shown in Table 6.1. There is no implication that variables not included in the model have in any way been demonstrated not to be associated with the outcomes reported. The results in Table 6.2 simply demonstrate those associations that dominated the variations in the outcome measures chosen. Stepwise regression analysis as a method of exploring the data is open to criticism in that the variables included may reflect chance associations discovered by estimating a series of mis-specified models. However, the theoretical implications of the inclusion and expected directions of influence have been closely monitored and the resulting set of equations presents a coherent and plausible set of hypotheses. The analysis of the residuals revealed no cause for concern, other than the effect of Centrelea on the analysis of the change in social disturbance. Even here examination of the domains of influence tended to reinforce the main messages of the model rather than suggest alternative influences at work.

Overall the results suggest that the supra-personal environment has an important effect on residents' behaviour and orientation. Higher turnover of residents was associated with increased social disturbance, but for both apathy and orientation staffing issues were of prime importance. These staffing influences can, perhaps, be summarised as availability, stability and training. The contrast in the effect of nursing qualifications on apathy and orientation is of particular interest, and the implications of this finding are discussed further in Chapter 7. Perhaps surprisingly, staffing issues were not found to impact directly on socially-disturbed behaviour.

The model described in Chapter 2 emphasised the importance of a resident's individual experience of the social and physical environmental effects, and the results in Chapter 3 indicate how much the individual experience can vary from the overall home environment. It is clear from the estimated model, however, that the overall environment does impact on residents. Positive regimes, the level of noise, and homes in which personal territory is of importance were all found to affect outcomes for residents. Additionally, individual levels of visiting, drugs and control were significant influences and the effect of residents' ability to find their way around is of particular interest given the results reported in Chapter 5. The next task is to examine the policy and practice implications of these results.

7 Policy implications and future research

While the current policy emphasis is on caring for people with all types of disability in the community, people with senile dementia present a number of difficulties to service providers. Their need for monitoring and the stress that they place on the people who care for them is such that residential care will often be the most appropriate type of care. Indeed, for people currently in long-term hospital wards, residential care represents a step towards 'care in the community'. Moreover, the policy impetus towards increasing choice and changing patterns of financial incentives, due to be introduced as a result of the *National Health Service and Community Care Act 1990*, mean that there will be added incentives to vary the ways in which 'shelter with care' (including all types of accommodation, from sheltered housing to nursing homes) is provided.

In monitoring the care of demented people, the role of the 'arms-length inspectorates' (Cm 849, 1989) will be of particular importance. People with dementia are even less able than other elderly residents to respond to low-quality care by leaving ('exiting') or complaining (exercising 'voice'): the main mechanisms by which falling standards are identified in the market place (Hirschmann, 1970). There will also be a need for an increased level of co-operation between health and social services agencies in order to ensure high-quality care for this particularly dependent group of people. Much has been written about the principles of good practice and care (Centre for Policy on Ageing, 1984; Wagner, 1988), but there is little direct evidence concerning the influences on the quality of life of demented elderly people in residential care. If the resources for monitoring and co-ordinating care for this group of people are to be properly targeted, there needs to be an increased level of understanding of the effects of residential care.

The underlying aim of the study reported here was to analyse the impact of the environment of homes for elderly people on the 'confused' resident. While the study was restricted to local authority homes, there is no reason to believe that the results should not apply to residential care provided by all sectors. Moreover, those features of the environment identified as associated with positive outcomes for residents can provide a basis for local authorities to monitor residential care of elderly people with senile dementia more effectively. The investigation was exploratory in approach, and the results should be seen only as a starting point for further research. However, it is of interest to explore the implications of the findings for policy, should they be confirmed in future work.

In Chapter 1 five areas of policy concern were identified in the field of residential care of demented elderly people: design; specialism; staffing; the role of residential homes in the community; and inspection, performance review and monitoring. The study was unusual in the UK research context in examining both the physical and the social environmental aspects of residential care. This chapter briefly discusses the need for future research before examining the policy and practice implications of the results of the study for each of these areas, and implications for innovative 'shelter with care'.

Research implications

In drawing out the possible policy implications of the study, there will be a tendency to draw inferences beyond the limits of validity. The whole exercise was intended to advance further certain hypotheses based on those in the literature and on associations found in a relatively small data set. A model based on the social ecology approach to the assessment of the environment has been used to aid this process and to describe the assumptions underlying the relationship between the environment and the resident. While the type of research design employed here has proved useful in describing the relationship between people with dementia and various aspects of the residential care environment, alternative approaches such as observation techniques would provide valuable insights into the nature of the relationships identified.

There are a great many directions in which future research can build on the findings of this study, but priorities in research depend on the implications for policy and practice in the future. Already a number of studies are building on the Wagner report in the form of the Residential Care Initiative and are developing such issues as training, performance and review, and complaints.

The results here suggest a number of other areas that would warrant further investigation and development. For example, given the current emphasis on the provision of support for carers, there is clearly a need for a comprehensive evaluation of relief care that takes into account the impact on the home as well as the recipient of the care. The results of this study also suggest that the characteristics of staff at homes for elderly people are of fundamental importance to the welfare of residents with senile dementia. Further work needs to be done to determine what issues affect staff sickness and turnover and the care staff to resident ratio that is required to ensure high-quality care when residents are 'confused'. It would be of immense value, moreover, to investigate further the nature of the staff/resident relationship, examining the strengths and weaknesses of the type of nursing qualifications and background of staff currently employed in residential care.

The regime measure could prove a useful tool for further research. The results reported here mirror the finding that resident well-being was significantly higher in homes that had the 'emergent-positive' social climate than in those with the 'open conflict' type of climate distinguished by Timko and Moos (1991). When examining the effects of treatments, such as reality orientation or activity programmes, the effect on staff morale has frequently been noted in the literature. Increased motivation and 'team spirit' among staff can result from such experiments and in turn affect the whole social 'atmosphere' or 'climate' of a ward or home. Monitoring the effect of such programmes on the overall social climate could, therefore, prove a useful device in analysing the relationship between 'Hawthorne effects' and the direct effect of the programmes.

There is considerable scope for validation of the measures and extension of the methods used to assess the physical environment. For example, route diagrams might be usefully extended and refined to assess other designs of homes. Validation of the 'Find' measure by observational work might result in a useful basis for comparing elderly people's ability to orientate themselves spatially in different environments. Further development of the methods and the establishment of normative data may allow assessments of the variation in the ways that designs of residential homes can affect elderly demented people. Furthermore, this study did not manage to establish any relationship between the use of orientation aids – such as colour-coding and large clear labelling – and residents' navigational abilities. An observation study on the 'Find' and 'route' measures may be able to assist in the development of a method for evaluating orientation aids.

The investigation of the physical environment highlighted the importance of relating outcomes for individual residents to both their individual experience of the homes and the overall design. It is clearly important not to assume that, as a stranger to a building, an alert individual will experience it in a similiar way to someone with short-term memory loss. Identifiable landmarks which provide aids to navigation are decision points which are used on a regular basis, not a specific design feature or an item such as an aquarium. Thus while it may make sense to suggest that people with dementia would benefit from designs in which they can see all the places they may need to use (dining area, WC and so on) from a single vantage point (Coles et al., 1992) such designs need to be evaluated in terms of outcomes for the residents themselves. It is plausible that such designs may overload residents with information so they cannot easily distinguish areas in the home they are looking for.

The results presented here do not simply provide pointers for future areas of investigation. They have implications for the future residential care of people with senile dementia. The following sections explore the findings further in the context of current developments in providing shelter with care.

Physical design of homes

The model on which the research was based emphasises the interactive nature of the relationship between people and their environments. Different aspects of the environment would also be expected to influence each other: the type of social climate that develops, for example, will be due in part to the type of building. In previous research some evidence has been found for a relationship between regime and the design of homes (Wyvern Partnership, 1979), but in this study the evidence is ambiguous: the 'restrictive' regimes included one home designed for group living and two purpose-built communal homes. Of the homes with 'positive' regimes, two were designed for group living and two were converted older buildings. Rather than contributing towards the generation of a 'positive' regime, it is more likely that those homes in older converted buildings which were clearly generating a 'positive' regime would be the last to be moved to more 'suitable' purpose-built premises.

One of the principal rationales for the group-living approach to residential care is that the groups offer the potential to develop individual social climates: 'family' lifestyles separate to that of the home at large (Norman, 1984). If this were occurring it would be expected that the social climate within these homes would vary between groups, but there was very little evidence of this in the separate assessments made by care staff in homes designed for group living. Mere physical organisation of people into distinguishable living areas is clearly not sufficient. Staff play a key role in the welfare of residents and while this influential population of the homes is not allocated to groups, the chances are that clearly-differentiated social climates are unlikely to develop. There was also no evidence of group-based activities which might have aided the development of a sense of cohesion or belonging.

The results of the study did suggest, however, that one advantage of group-living designs was being exploited: the enabling of residents to restrict their use of the home so they could maximise their ability to negotiate their environment. While desirable in its own right, the ability to navigate the home was also found to be associated with changes in levels of apathy and contentedness in residents. In social ecological terms, the need to get to a single dining area in homes designed for communal living resulted in increased environmental press with regard to residents' physical competence. Allowing some residents to eat away from the main dining rooms, so their 'route' can be limited to one section of the home if they desire, may be one way of aiding a resident to cope with such designs. In group-living homes attention to the level of lighting and placing residents in bedrooms on corridor junctions are likely to help residents find their way around.

While lighting was key to people finding their way around the home, the level of noise was directly associated with behavioural and orientation outcomes. As Wightman (1992) points out, provision for adequate noise insulation is often a victim of cost-cutting. While there are ways in which staff can reduce noise levels in a home, the acoustic quality of harsh reverberant interiors may negate such attempts. Interior design and furnishings which reduce reverberation are clearly desirable in the light of the effect of noise on people with dementia.

Evidence about the importance of territorial issues in the homes is thin but of interest. The size of bedroom areas in some cases was extremely small (two square metres in one case), far below recommended levels (Department of Health and Social Security, 1973). If the association between bedroom size and territorial behaviour by residents (in the form of 'own' chairs) and between this and lower levels of contentment proves causal, this would lend weight to the argument that personal territory is an important issue for residents with confusional problems.

It has been argued that one way of clearly establishing territory is through personalising an area with possessions. In the homes in the study, bedrooms very rarely appeared to 'belong' to residents. Often fewer personal possessions were in evidence than might be seen in short-term hospital wards. The absence of effects associated with well-established territory may reflect the very low levels which prevailed generally. The policy of allowing residents to bring in furniture is clearly not enough. The emphasis needs to shift to an understanding that residents will furnish their rooms and that furniture will be provided if they do not have anything suitable. Only in this way can residents feel that this is their home. There are no better 'multiple cues' to a bedroom than long-established possessions. There are increasingly calls for single rooms with en suite toilet facilities to be provided as standard (Coles et al., 1992). Such provision may also serve to enhance a sense of territory.

There was no evidence that people with dementia have requirements of the design of homes that are incompatible with those of people without mental difficulties. While the need to have an easily-understood environment for navigation purposes is clearly less for such residents, the finding that communal-living homes make residents with physical disabilities unnecessarily dependent on staff is equally applicable. Similarly the needs of mentally alert residents for adequate private space has been well-documented in the literature (for example, Willcocks et al., 1987) and it is not surprising that lack of such space should be associated, however indirectly, with contendedness for residents with confusional difficulties. Moreover, where homes were purpose-built for the care of elderly people with mental infirmity, they were as likely to be associated with a restrictive regime as with a positive one.

Specialist provision

One small-scale study in the USA (Rovner et al., 1990) contrasted outcomes for residents in a special unit with those in the rest of a nursing home and found that the functional capacity of the residents of the unit remained stable while the control group deteriorated. Necessarily, given the research design, the results from this study are much less clear-cut. The specialist facilities in the study included a wide variety of establishments and there was no consistent relationship with beneficial outcomes for residents and specialism among the homes. However, some of the results would imply the increased use of specialist resources, perhaps joint provision with health authorities as recommended in Wagner (1988, p.117). Specialist homes have higher staffing levels and should ideally be able to draw on expert sources that prevent overprescription of drugs, although the variety of homes included as specialist in this study did not show this latter trait consistently. Specialist homes, however, did have significantly higher SCES scores for cohesion, self-disclosure and independence and were significantly quieter. Moreover, while it is neither necessary nor sufficient for a home to be specialist to achieve a 'positive' regime, it can provide a basis for a distinctive home philosophy which encourages this.

Demographic and policy pressures are such that inevitably non-specialist homes will need to care for people with confusional difficulties. The pressures that these residents put on homes are such that there is a need for specialist knowledge about the care of people with dementia in all homes that are prepared to admit people with confusional difficulties. One way of dealing with this is to attach a specialist unit with higher staff-resident ratios for people with confusional difficulties to a non-specialist home, and it was noted in the Wagner Review (1988) that there was an increased tendency for homes to have such units. Lodge (1991) recommends this type of approach on the basis that it provides opportunities to mix with other groups and types of people. Moreover, if the use of specialist units resulted in a greater dispersal of provision of places, it could make visiting easier for relatives and friends. It is probable, however, that units attached to homes would need to be carefully staffed and treated very much as a separate entity to the rest of the home if there was to be a chance of the 'positive' type of regime being generated.

In all homes caring for people with senile dementia, specialist knowledge about the importance of issues such as the effect of noise on demented residents enables good practice to be adopted – for example, limiting the use of televisions to specific areas, and controlling the degree to which residents distract one another by taking loud residents for timely walks. Pressures on staff can result in more restrictive practices with such residents, especially where the 'common sense' option might appear to minimise risk. The evidence here suggests that residents with very limited control need to retain all possible control over their daily lives.

Staffing

Specialist knowledge in the form of nursing qualifications already exists in many homes. The results presented here suggest that this is a two-edged sword, however. Among those concerned with the residential care of people with senile dementia, there needs to be an awareness that staff who are recruited to homes for elderly people may have the type of nursing background that leads them to fail to respond to the problem of apathy among the residents. While in-service training is not clearly associated with positive outcomes for residents, it has a vital role to play in building on the strengths and mitigating the disadvantages of such backgrounds. The only specific type of training recommended by the Wagner Review (1988) was in social work. The lack of evidence of a direct relationship with client outcomes is probably primarily due to the low incidence of such qualifications: in the homes as a whole only 5 per cent of care and supervisory staff had any type of social work qualification.

One of the messages of most immediate concern to staff in the field of residential care of demented elderly people is the importance of their own role. The need for adequate staffing, low turnover and for the involvement and commitment of staff in the care of demented residents cannot be over-emphasised. These factors have a direct impact on the residents, reducing apathy and encouraging orientation. There was also an indirect effect: through the influence of homes with positive regimes. At first sight the four homes (Pondlea, Haddock House, Chaucer Place and Westgate) were very different, yet one feature that did link the four was the high level of involvement and status of the care staff.

Three of the homes with positive regimes were specialist establishments. In one there were no 'care assistants', only 'residential social workers' and 'assistant residential social workers'. This home had a vast throughput of agency staff (74 different people in six months!) because adequate staffing levels were seen as essential. In two of the other homes the keyworker schemes were active and used: the care staff concerned were consulted and involved in this study wherever possible. In one of these homes the management was so devolved that the researcher never wittingly met the officer-in-charge. In the other the officer-in-charge was responsible for a large proportion of the training of care assistants in caring for demented people in the local authority. In all three of these homes a heavy emphasis was laid on the training and involvement of care staff.

The fourth home was non-specialist, but again involved the staff and anybody who visited the home in its extensive social life. Visitors and the local community were drawn into the home and staff often would bring their families to the social events. Pride was taken in the achievements of residents; on the researcher's arrival at the home one lady was introduced who had learned to knit while in the home. It did not appear to matter, therefore, whether the dominant philosophy of the home was reality orientation or community involvement. What was important was that there *was* a dominant philosophy in which care staff were perceived, and perceived themselves, to be an essential ingredient.

Overall, the message for staff is that their availability, stability and motivation are key ingredients in providing high-quality care for residents with senile dementia. Staff themselves find the experience of insufficient staff on duty as stressful (Benjamin and Spector, 1990b) and this is particularly likely to be the case where there is a high level of sickness and a high turnover of staff. High levels of stress can lead to higher levels of sickness and staff leaving and the problem becomes self-perpetuating. Clearly, however, such vicious circles can be broken through specific initiatives to increase staffing levels and through training. The evidence from this study suggests that residents directly benefit from resulting 'virtuous circles' of adequate staffing levels, high motivation, low levels of stress, less sickness and lower staff turnover.

Role of facilities in the community

A high turnover of residents as well as staff was found to have an adverse effect on residents. High turnover of residents resulted in higher levels of social disturbance among the sample residents and was associated with the provision of rotating or respite care. Moreover, there is evidence that the 'disruptive' effect of short-term care suggested by *Home Life* (Centre for Policy on Ageing, 1984) does indeed occur and prevents the formation of positive supportive regimes. This supports the findings by others (for example, Kuh and Boldy, 1981; Allen, 1983; Morton, 1991) that permanent, alert, residents reject short-stay residents.

The provision of respite care is likely to become of increasing concern in the future in order to provide support for the growing number of demented people being cared for in the community (Levin et al., 1989). These results suggest that how this is provided is of the utmost importance to permanent residents with senile dementia. There may be an argument for separating relief care entirely from long-stay care for demented residents, both physically and in service terms. Thus certain establishments would specialise in rotating care and relief care schemes, and residential care homes would provide permanent care. In practice, officers-in charge will be under pressure to use spare capacity for the provision of short-term care, and case managers to find places wherever they are available. In such circumstances the impact of turnover of residents might be minimised as far as possible by, for example, limiting short-term care to one group in group-living homes

Keeping links with the community so homes do not become socially marooned' is clearly of importance. Visitors to residents are one of the strongest connections with the community and have been found to be associated here with maintaining residents' levels of orientation. Relatives and friends provide links with the past and also a level of individual stimulation that can be difficult for staff to provide. The amount relatives and friends can visit will largely be determined by the location of the home, although staff have a vital role to play in supporting relatives who may find the process of visiting distressing and/or discouraging.

Inspection, performance review and the monitoring role of local authorities

One approach to monitoring the quality of care suggests three types of criteria: structure, process and outcome (Donabedian, 1982). 'Structure' refers to resources used and the stable arrangements under which care is produced. In the case of residential care, this would include an indicator of the number of beds in a home. 'Process' refers to activities that constitute care, such as caring regimes and management style for example. 'Outcomes' are the consequences for the health or welfare of the client, such as morbidity or quality of life. Inspection and performance review are concerned with assessing the process of care. The most direct route is to evaluate the process itself, but in practice issues of structure are easier to identify and to measure.

In *Homes Are For Living In*, the Social Services Inspectorate (DH/SSI, 1989a) argued for more emphasis on assessing quality of care and less on such structural issues as building standards, staffing arrangements and record-keeping. They proposed that the factors that contribute to quality centre on six basic values: privacy, dignity, independence, choice, rights and fulfilment. One of the underlying reasons for poor practice, however, is not disagreement about these underlying values but inappropriate responses to conflict between the aims of residential care. Much stress is laid in residential care on the physical safety of residents, but the placing of fire doors can directly conflict with residents' need for independence in terms of free movement around the home. If confused elderly people have problems getting themselves dressed, is it more important that they retain the independence and choice to wear a peculiar assortment of clothes or the dignity of being dressed as they were before the onset of dementia? Clearly the question is one of balance between such issues, and evaluating whether the right balance is found is the concern of those who set out to inspect or review the performance of a home. It is necessary in inspection and monitoring, therefore, to be aware of the relationship between the caring process, outcomes for residents, and the structure within which care is provided.

The results reported here identify a number of measures that are likely to influence the welfare of elderly people with confusional difficulties: the design of the home, staffing ratios, turnover, sickness and so on. But the existence of appropriate policies on choice, for example, cannot be taken as an indicator of appropriate process in the care of demented elderly people. Clark and Bowling (1990) found that relatively invariant measures of regime concealed a wide variety of care practices when qualitative techniques of assessment were used. Moreover, in the study reported here, judgements about residents' competence affected whether they were offered choice over clothes. The fact that this in turn was associated with socially-disturbed behaviour suggests that inappropriate limitations on choice affect residents' welfare.

Another process issue raised by the study is the use of psychotropic drugs in homes for elderly people. In particular, it is of concern that the policy in which a home is allocated a GP, with whom most residents are registered, did not appear to translate into more careful prescribing of drugs. There have already been a number of investigations (for example, Wade et al., 1986) which have voiced concern at the use of drugs in the care of elderly people in residential care. The results of this study would indicate that, in adopting a monitoring role, local authorities will need to establish clear and enforceable guidelines which ensure that expert medical supervision is available and used by all homes caring for people with senile dementia.

The association between the homes with 'positive' regimes and three of the outcome measures used, if confirmed by future research, could provide the basis for an evaluative tool in providing a link between measures of process in residential care and outcome for residents with confusional states. If further research established a link between positive regimes and beneficial outcomes for alert elderly people, such an application could be usefully widened. For example, Gibbs and Sinclair (1991) found that using the checklist approach to inspection produced a very low level of agreement among inspectors, particularly of local authority homes. An alternative method of assessing the social environment could be used to analyse the reasons for this and provide a basis for comparing the validity of different checklists.

As it stands the SCES scale would be rather unwieldy for use in the inspection process itself or for the self-monitoring of homes. It may prove possible to adapt the approach (Fyvie and Gledhill, 1989), but even as it stands it offers a basis for evaluating other tools and approaches such as identifying desirable characteristics of heads of homes which are crucial to the quality of an establishment (Gibbs and Sinclair, 1991). It is particularly useful in identifying positive aspects of the residential care environment. If the Wagner principle that residential care should be a positive choice is to become a reality, the emphasis when monitoring homes must on quality assurance rather than primarily inspecting for faults.

Innovations in residential care of people with dementia

In Chapter 1 it was demonstrated that as a result of population changes there was likely to be a continuing if not a growing need for residential care for people with senile dementia. Even with the most determined policy of providing care in people's own homes, this will leave a role for residential care for those with confusional problems. In Denmark there has been legislation to prevent the building of any more residential nursing homes, with the intention that elderly people in need of extensive care should be placed in their own independent homes in small congregate housing projects (Frickmann, 1991). These projects would cater for a range of ages but it has been acknowledged that there would be limits to the degree to which they could cater for people with senile dementia, and the existing residential nursing homes may well make up the expected shortfall in specialist accomodation (Frickmann, 1991).

There is a growing number of variations, however, in the way that residential care of people with senile dementia is being provided. In Sweden, group-living units, which consist of flats in ordinary blocks, are being used for the care of demented residents. These are staffed 24 hours a day with specially trained staff (Wimo et al., 1991). While there are limitations on the types of disabilities that can be catered for, the results of an evaluation suggest that a better quality of life can be obtained at a lower cost than would have been incurred in an ordinary nursing home or on a hospital ward. Certainly the emphasis on staff motivation and the small, domestic scale nature of the design fit in well with the results of the study reported on here.

Lodge (1990) has reviewed developments in British residential care of people with dementia. He suggests that there are three basic desirable types of accommodation which cover the range of needs of people with dementia: high, medium and low health input care homes. High health care input schemes are demonstrated by developments in modifying NHS nursing homes. Medium health input care is reflected by developments in social services group homes, and low health input by 'the modified housing with extra care' style of scheme. In each case the emphasis is on small groups of residents and each of the examples cited was characterised by a clear philosophy of care often developed and supported by multidisciplinary teams or advisory groups. Some new developments have focused on the flexible use of establishments, providing a range of services, day and respite care as well as permanent beds (Donaldson and Gregson, 1988; Pattie and Moxon, 1991). While there is evidence that these are effective in maintaining people longer in the community (Donaldson and Gregson, 1989), there is little direct evidence of the effect of this type of establishment on permanent residents. The results from this study would suggest that this type of establishment would be disruptive to permanent residents although orientation might be maintained at a higher level as a result of higher carer involvement.

The domus, a small-scale NHS-managed residential unit, has a philosophy of care which addresses 'staff anxieties and attitudes that lead to institutional maintenance and poor quality of life for residents' (Lindesay et al., 1991, p.728). Clearly this philosophy is aimed at the heart of the problem of balancing the conflicting objectives of residential care identified above. It is based on four assumptions:

- that the domus is the residents' home for life;
- that the needs of the staff are as important as those of the residents;
- that the domus should aim to correct the avoidable consequences of dementia and accommodate those that are unavoidable; and
- that the residents' individual psychological and emotional needs may take precedence over the physical aspects of care (Lindesay et al., 1991, p.728).

The results of the investigation reported here support this philosophy and many other current developments in residential care. Reservations have been expressed, however, about the 'practicality' of the domus (Lodge, 1990), primarily because of the extremely high costs involved (Beecham et al., 1991). Indeed, cost is likely to be the stumbling block to the growing consensus about what constitutes good quality care. Small groups with high levels of staffing and multidisciplinary inputs are not cheap options. The care of people with senile dementia, more than any other group, will put to the test just what is considered 'value for money' under the new legislation (Cm 849, 1989). This makes it all the more important that there are good data on the structure, processes and outcomes of different care environments.

The model used as the basis for the study described here suggests that another fundamental aim of the legislation – to improve consumer choice – will feed directly into this 'value-for-money' issue. Different types of care environment will suit or 'fit' different individuals: the more variety of types of care on offer, the greater the possibility there is of finding the best type of environment for the circumstances of any given individual. This raises the question of whether the results of this study when put in the context of other research findings suggest any new developments in the field of residential care of people with senile dementia.

One possible way forward that builds on developments such as the domus, the findings here and research in the field of informal care of people with confusional difficulties, is the concept of 'informal care homes'.

Informal care homes

In investigating the effect of the environment of homes on residents with senile dementia there has been no attempt to contrast the outcomes with those that would have been obtained if people had remained in their own homes. The point has repeatedly been made that there are limits to the degree that maintaining people with senile dementia in community is possible and the focus of interest has been on the most beneficial or positive environment in the residential care setting. This is of particular importance to relatives when residential care becomes an issue. They need to know that the move will be for the best for the elderly person concerned. Clearly, however, in many cases the best option for the elderly person will be to stay at home, in a small domestic setting with an intensive one-to-one long-term care relationship. It is an acknowledgement of this fact, among other things, that leads many people to continue to care until they are highly stressed and can cope no longer (Argyle, 1985). Thus it is carers' attitude rather than disability that is the principal predictor of entry into institutional care (Levin et al., 1983; Lieberman and Kramer, 1991).

The belief that the welfare of the elderly person is best served by remaining at home is not the only reason that relatives continue to care in situations of great strain. When people are sharing households, the income of an additional pension and other allowances can make a substantial contribution to household finances not entirely offset by the costs of providing care. Moreover, carers often develop skills in the process of caring which will be lost. The more their lives have become constrained by the caring role, the more they will be giving up an investment in their own development and losing an important dimension to their own lives. This situation does not apply to all carers, but a substantial proportion of primary carers are spouses and the pressures to continue to care in spite of health and social care needs of their own are particularly high in this group (Pollitt et al., 1991).

This conflict in needs between carers and the cared for and increasing emphasis on supporting carers has accelerated developments in providing breaks or respite care to enable carers to carry on caring at home (Levin and Moriarty, 1990). These take the form of relief care in homes, day care, sitting services and a limited number of family placements and overnight respite schemes. By far the most widespread of these is day care. While the benefit derived by carers from these services is considerable, the degree to which respite care actually substitutes for admitting elderly people with dementia into long-term residential care appears limited (Levin et al., 1992). Often acceptance of relief care is a precursor to long-term admission rather than an alternative.

Services which are intended to bring relief and to support carers are based on the assumption that the bulk of care will continue to be provided by the carer at home. In addition there is an assumption that on admission the carers' problems will disappear, although there is evidence that admission of demented relatives long-term residential care does not always result in reduced stress among carers (Stephens et al., 1991; Levin et al., 1992). Lewis and Meredith (1989), in discussing conflicts between informal and formal care, reported that many carers' sense of self-worth was interwoven with the activity of caring. This can make the transition to residential care particularly difficult.

An alternative approach would be to provide a residential facility staffed to provide weekend and night care for the elderly person in a small establishment (with the small domestic scale of the domus) close to the carer's home. The carer, however, would continue to be the 'keyworker' and retain prime responsibility for providing care at the establishment for the elderly person during the day. They could reduce their involvement from the 24 hours required in their own home to, for example, a five day week. The actual level of involvement would be negotiable but the emphasis would be on building on the experience and skills of the carer in caring for their relative. This approach would reduce the tremendous waste of knowledge and expertise that occurs when the carer gives up the principal caring role to an establishment. Professional staff would be available for advice and support but the way in which the informal care home developed would depend on the needs of the carers and the elderly people being cared for. This would reduce the need for an 'all or nothing' decision on the part of the carer who could also gain from and provide support to other carers in the home.

Such an approach could provide the high, consistent level of staffing shown in this study to be beneficial; the familiarity provided by regular visits and the small domestic scale would contribute to the residents' ability to find their way around and to a quiet atmosphere. The input from professional staff could enable monitoring of drug use and encourage appropriate care practices based on the domus philosophy and a 'positive' regime. The carers could retain their primary role but lead a more normal life, assured of a lack of disruption at night and at the weekends, thus allowing the possibility of rebuilding their own lives without having to give up their commitment to the elderly person. Central to the concept would be flexibility. Some homes may make very few demands on professionals; others may develop into traditional but small-scale residential homes with a low input from carers. Professional support should ensure that the informal care home can support people with very high levels of disability, so there would be no need to leave the home other than for acute hospital care. While the expectation would not be that carers would be paid a full wage, continued eligibility for attendance allowance or some type of payment for their continued involvement might reduce the financial impact of the elderly person leaving the household on the carer. From the perspective of the providing agency, a much higher level of care could be obtained for the costs of providing the informal care home than would be possible in mainstream residential or nursing home care.

This type of scheme would not be appropriate for those carers who wish to return to or continue with waged work or those with other commitments. But it may provide an alternative to those relatives who live in separate households and cannot or do not wish to share a household with the elderly person and who wish to continue to care for a relative who needs more support at home than domiciliary services can provide. Informal care homes probably have a very small role to play in aiding carers and elderly people to make the transition from private households to accommodation-based care and any development clearly would need to be preceded by a detailed investigation into the likely demand for such a service. But such an approach could allow greater flexibility in the type of commitment carers need to make and would increase the diversity of options available.

Conclusion

While such innovations may be useful, they will inevitably play a minor role in the continuing care of people with dementia. Mainstream residential and nursing home provision will continue to have a major role to play, however. The study reported here was small in scale and there are limitations on the conclusions that can be drawn, but it is hoped that this will prove a useful contribution to a specific area which contains very little in the way of research that relates measures of outcomes for demented residents to the experience of residential care.

Booth concluded from his investigations into residential care for elderly people that

> Whatever factors account for the variations in outcome between homes seem to be outside the immediate control of the staff (Booth, 1986, p.235).

The results of this study, if confirmed, challenge this pessimistic conclusion. Many of the influences found to be of importance for outcomes of elderly demented people are well within the control of staff, given sufficient motivation and resources. The conflicting needs of elderly people with confusional difficulties mean that providing good quality care will always be a balancing act, but one that it is clearly possible to accomplish.

References

Allen, I. (1983) *Short-Stay Residential Care for the Elderly*, Policy Studies Institute, London.

Allen, I. (1986) Short stay residential care and other uses of local authority homes for the elderly, in K. Judge and I. Sinclair (eds) *Residential Care for Elderly People*, HMSO, London.

American Psychiatric Association (1980) *Diagnostic and Statistical Manual of Mental Disorders*, 3rd edition, American Psychiatric Association, Washington, D.C.

Anderson, J. (1990) The TAPS project: I. Previous psychiatric diagnosis and current disability of long-stay psychogeriatric patients, *British Journal of Psychiatry*, 156, 661-70.

Arber, S. and Ginn, J. (1990) The meaning of informal care: gender and the contribution of elderly people, *Ageing and Society*, 10, 429-54.

Argyle, N., Jestice, S., Brook, C. (1985) Psychogeriatric patients: their supporters' problems, *Age and Ageing*, 14, 355-360.

Arie, T. and Jolley, D. (1982) Making services work, in R. Levy and F. Post (eds) *The Psychiatry of Later Life*, Blackwell Scientific Publications, Oxford.

Atkinson, D., Bond, J. and Gregson, B. (1986) The dependency characteristics of older people in long term institutional care, in C. Phillipson, M. Bernard and P. Strang (eds) *Dependency and Interdependency in Old Age – Theoretical Perspectives and Policy Alternatives*, Croom Helm, London.

Barclay, P. (1982) *Social Workers, their Roles and Tasks*, Institute for Social Work, Bedford Square Press, London.

Barton, R. (1966) *Institutional Neurosis*, 2nd edition, Wright, Bristol.

Beecham, J., Cambridge, P., Hallam, A. and Knapp, M.R.J. (1991) The costs of domus care in Lewisham, Discussion Paper 774, Personal Social Services Research Unit, University of Kent at Canterbury.

Benjamin, L. and Spector, J. (1990a) Environments for the dementing, *International Journal of Geriatric Psychiatry*, 5, 15-24.

Benjamin, L. and Spector, J. (1990b) The relationship of staff, resident and environmental characteristics to stress experienced by staff caring for the dementing, *International Journal of Geriatric Psychiatry*, 5, 25-31.

Bergmann, K., Foster, E., Justice, A., Matthews, V. (1978) Management of the demented elderly patient in the community, *British Journal of Psychiatry*, 132, 441-9.

Bergmann, K. and Jacoby, R. (1982) The limitations and possibilities of community care for the elderly demented, in Department of Health and Social Security (ed.) *Elderly People in the Community: Their Service Needs*, HMSO, London.

Berkman, L. and Syme, S. (1979) Social networks, host resistance and mortality: a nine year follow up of Aldmeda country residents, *American Journal of Epidemiology*, 109, 186-204.

Blenkner, M. (1967), Environmental change and the aging individual, *The Gerontologist*, 7, 2, 101-5.

Bond, J., Bond, S., Donaldson, C., Gregson, B. and Atkinson, A. (1989) Evaluation of an innovation in the continuing care of very frail elderly people, *Ageing and Society*, 9, 4, 347-82.

Booth, T. (1983) The rising tide, *Community Care*, 10 March, 23-5.

Booth, T. (1985) *Home Truths: Old Peoples Homes and the Outcome of Care*, Gower, Aldershot.

Booth, T. (1986) Institutional regimes and induced dependency in homes for the aged, *The Gerontologist*, 26, 4, 418-23.

Calkins, M.P. (1988) *Design for Dementia: Planning Environments for the Elderly and the Confused*, National Health Publishing, Owings Mills, Maryland.

Centre for Policy on Ageing (1984) *Home Life: A Code of Practice for Residential Care*, Centre for Policy on Ageing, London.

Challis, D.J. (1981) The measurement of outcome in social care of the elderly, *Journal of Social Policy*, 10, 2, 179-208.

Challis, D.J. and Davies, B.P. (1986) *Case Management in Community Care*, Gower, Aldershot.

Christie, A. (1985) Survival in dementia: a review, in T. Arie (ed.) *Recent Advances in Psychogeriatrics*, Churchill Livingstone, Edinburgh.

Clark, P. and Bowling, A. (1990) Quality of everyday life in long stay institutions for the elderly: an observational study of long stay hospital and nursing home care, *Social Science and Medicine*, 30, 11, 1201-10.

Clarke, M., Lowry, R. and Clarke, S. (1986) Cognitive impairment in the elderly: a community survey, *Age and Ageing*, 5, 278-84.

Clough, R. (1981) *Old Age Homes*, Allen and Unwin, London.

Cm 849 (1989) *Caring for People*, HMSO, London.

Coles, R., Duncan, I., Kelly, M., Marshall, M. and Wightman, A. (eds)(1992) *Signposts Not Barriers*, Dementia Services Development Centre, University of Stirling.

Cox, P. (1990) Care for elderly mentally ill people: a special market niche presentation of elderly care prospects for the 1990s, given at a conference organised by Laing & Buisson and Healthcare Information Services, March, London.

Cummings, E., Dean, L., Newall, D., McCaffrey, I. (1972) Disengagement: a tentative theory of ageing, in S. Chown (ed.) *Human Ageing*, Penguin Books, Harmondsworth.

Darton, R. (1983) Residential accommodation for the elderly, 1970-81, PSSRU Discussion Paper 277/2, Personal Social Services Research Unit, University of Kent at Canterbury.

Darton, R. (1986a) Methodological report of the PSSRU survey of residential accommodation for the elderly, 1981, PSSRU Discussion Paper 422, Personal Social Services Research Unit, University of Kent at Canterbury.

Darton, R. (1986b) PSSRU survey of residential accommodation for the elderly, 1981. Characteristics of the residents, PSSRU Discussion Paper 426, Personal Social Services Research Unit, University of Kent at Canterbury.

Darton, R. and Wright, K. (1989) PSSRU/CHE survey of residential and nursing homes: preliminary information on the characteristics of homes and residents and patients in non-statutory homes, and comparisons with the public sector, PSSRU Discussion Paper 617, Personal Social Services Research Unit, University of Kent at Canterbury.

Davies, B.P. and Knapp, M.R.J. (1981) *Old Peoples' Homes and the Production of Welfare*, Routledge and Kegan Paul, London.

De Long, A. (1974) Environments for the elderly, *Journal of Communications*, 24, 4, 101-2.

Department of Health and Social Security (1973) *Residential Accommodation for the Elderly*, Local Authority Building Note number 2, HMSO, London.

Department of Health and Social Security (1977) *Residential Homes for the Elderly: Arrangements for Health Care, A Memorandum of Guidance*, Department of Health and Social Security, London.

Department of Health and Social Security (1981) *Growing Older*, HMSO, London.

Department of Health/Social Services Inspectorate (1989a) *Homes are for Living In*, HMSO, London.

Department of Health/Social Services Inspectorate (1989b) *Towards a Climate of Confidence*, HMSO, London.

Department of Health/Social Services Inspectorate (1991) *Caring for Quality: Guidance on Standards for Residential Homes for Elderly People*, HMSO, London.

Donabedian, A. (1982) *The Criteria and Standards of Quality*, Health Administration Press, Ann Arbor, Michigan.

Donaldson, C. and Gregson, B. (1989) Prolonging life at home: what is the cost? *Community Medicine*, 2, 3, 200-209.

Evans, G., Hughes, B. and Wilkin, D. (1980) Issues in residential care of the elderly, research report, University Hospital of South Manchester Psychogeriatric Unit, Manchester.

Evans, G., Hughes, B., Wilkin, D. and Jolley, D. (1981) The management of mental and physical impairment in non-specialist residential homes for the elderly, research report, University Hospital of South Manchester Psychogeriatric Unit, Manchester.

Everitt, B. (1980) *Cluster Analysis*, 2nd edition, Heinemann, London.

Feier, C. and Leight, G. (1981) A communication-cognition program for elderly nursing home residents, *The Gerontologist*, 21, 4, 408-16.

Feil, N. (1985) Resolution: the final life task, *Journal of Humanistic Psychology*, 25, 2, 91-105.

Felce, D. and Jenkins, J. (1979) Engagement in activities by old people in residential care, *Health and Social Service Journal*, 2 November.

Frickmann, K.O. (1991) Social housing and care schemes for elderly people, in Royal Surgical Aid Society Symposium *Building and Designing for the Frail Elderly*, Royal Surgical Aid Society, London.

Fries, J.F. (1989) The compression of morbidity: near or far? *The Milbank Quarterly*, 67, 2, 208-32.

Fyvie, C. and Gledhill, K.J. (1989) Measuring staff perceptions of residential care settings for the elderly, paper presented to the British Society of Gerontology conference, Nottingham.

Garibaldi, R.A., Brodine, R.N. and Matsumiya, R.N. (1981) Infections among patients in nursing homes, *New England Journal of Medicine*, 305, 731-5.

Gibbs, I. and Sinclair, I. (1991) A checklist approach to the inspection of old people's homes, final report to the Department of Health, Department of Social Policy and Social Work, University of York.

Gilhooly, M. (1984) The social dimension of senile dementia, in I. Hanley and J. Hodge (eds) *Psychological Approaches to the Care of the Elderly*, Methuen, London.

Gilleard, C. (1982) Stresses and strains amongst supporters of the elderly infirm day hospital attenders, unpublished interim report, Psychogeriatric Day Centre Research Project, Department of Psychiatry, University of Edinburgh.

Gilleard, C. (1989) Losing one's mind and losing one's place: a psycho-social model of dementia, paper presented to British Society of Gerontology conference, Nottingham.

Goffman, E. (1961) *Asylums: Essays on the Social Situation of Mental Patients and other Inmates*, Doubleday, New York.

Gray, B. and Isaacs, B. (1979) *Care of the Elderly Mentally Infirm*, Tavistock Publications, London.

Green, W. (1989) *Buildings for the Neighbourhood Care of Elderly People with Dementia*, Help the Aged, London.

Griffiths, R. (1988) *Community Care: Agenda for Action*, HMSO, London.

Hagnell, O., Lanke, J., Rorsman, B., Ohman, R. and Ojesjo, L. (1981) Does the incidence of age psychosis decrease? A prospective, longitudinal study of the complete population investigated during the 25-year period 1947-1972; the Lundby study, *Neuropsychobiology*, 7, 201-11.

Hamilton, M. (1960) A rating scale for depression, *Journal of Neurology, Neurosurgery and Psychiatry*, 23, 56-62.

Harris, H. and Lipman, A. (1980) Social symbolism and space usage in daily life, *Sociological Review* 28, 2, 415-28.

Harris, H., Lipman, A., Slater, R. (1977) Architectural design: the spatial location and interaction of old people, *Gerontology*, 23, 390-400.

Harrison, R., Savla, N. and Kafetz, K. (1990) Dementia, depression and physical disability in a London borough: a survey of elderly people in and out of residential care and implications for future developments, *Age and Ageing*, 19, 97-103.

Health Advisory Service (1982) *The Rising Tide: Developing Services for Mental Illness in Old Age*, Health Advisory Service, London.

Henderson, A. (1986) The epidemiology of Alzheimer's Disease, *British Medical Bulletin*, 42, 1, 3-10.

Henwood, M. and Wicks, M. (1984) *The Forgotten Army*, Family Policy Studies Centre, London.

Hirschfeld, M. (1978) Families living with senile brain disease, dissertation submitted in partial satisfaction of the requirements of Doctor of Nursing Science, University of California, San Francisco.

Hirschmann, A. (1970) *Exit, Voice and Loyalty*, Harvard University Press, Cambridge, Massachusetts.

Hofman, A., Rocca, W., Brayne, C., Breteler, M., Clarke, M., Cooper, B., Copeland, J., Dartiques, J., de Silva Droux, A., Hagnell, O., Heeren, T., Engedal, K., Jonker, C., Lindsay, J., Lobo, A., Mann, A., Molsa, P., Morgan, K., O'Connor, D., Sulkava, R., Kay, D. and Amaducci, L. (1991) The prevalence of dementia in Europe, *International Journal of Epidemiology*, 20, 736-45.

Holden, U. and Woods, R. (1982) *Reality Orientation: Psychological Approaches to the 'Confused' Elderly*, Churchill Livingstone, Edinburgh.

Ineichen, B. (1987) Measuring the rising tide: how many dementia cases will there be by 2001? *British Journal of Psychiatry*, 150, 193-200.

Jenkins, J., Felce, D., Powell, E. and Lunt, B. (1977) Measuring client engagement in residential settings for the elderly, Research Report 120, Health Care Evaluation Team, Wessex Regional Health Authority, Winchester.

Jöreskog, K. and Sörbom, D. (1986) *LISREL Users Guide*, University of Uppsala, Sweden.

Jorm, A.F., Korten, A.E. and Henderson, A.S. (1987) The prevalence of dementia: a quantitative integration of the literature, *Acta Psychiatr Scand*, 76, 465-79.

Kahana, E. (1982) A conscience model of person environment interaction, in M. Lawton, P. Windley and T. Byerts (eds) *Aging and the Theoretical Approaches*, Springer, New York.

Kane, R. and Kane, R. (1981) *Assessing the Elderly. A Practical Guide to Measurement*, Lexington Books, Lexington, Massachusetts.

Kay, D., Beamish, P. and Roth, M. (1964) Old age mental disorders in Newcastle-Upon-Tyne: Part I, A study of prevalence, and Part II. A study of possible social and medical causes, *British Journal of Psychiatry*, 110, 146-59 and 668-82.

Kay, D., Bergman, K., Foster E., McKechnie, A. and Roth, M. (1970) Mental illness and hospital usage in the elderly: a random sample follow up, *Comprehensive Psychiatry*, 11, 20-35.

Keen, J. (1989) Interiors: architecture in the lives of people with dementia, *International Journal of Geriatric Psychiatry*, 4, 255-72.
Kellaher, L. (1986) Determinants of quality of life in residential settings for old people, in K. Judge and I. Sinclair (eds) *Residential Care for Elderly People*, HMSO, London.
Kimbell, A., Townsend, J. and Bird, M. (1974) Elderly persons' homes: a study of various aspects of regime and activities in elderly persons' homes and their effect upon residents, mimeograph, Cheshire Social Services Department, Chester.
King, R., Raynes, N., Tizard, J. (1971) *Patterns of Residential Care*, Routledge and Kegan Paul, London.
Kirby, H. and Harper, R. (1988) Team assessment of geriatric mental patients (II): Behavioural dynamics and psychometric testing in the diagnosis of functional dementia due to hysterical behaviour, *The Gerontologist*, 28, 2, 260-62.
Knapp, M.R.J. (1984) *The Economics of Social Care*, Macmillan, London.
Korte, S. (1966) Designing for old people: the role of residential homes, *The Architectural Journal*, 19 October, 987-91.
Kraan, R.J., Baldock, J., Davies, B.P., Evers, A., Johansson, L., Knapen, M., Thorslund, M. and Tunissen, C. (1991) *Care for the Elderly: Significant Innovations in Three European Countries*, European Centre for Social Welfare Policy and Research, Frankfurt am Main and Campus/Westview, Boulder, Colorado.
Kuh, D. and Boldy, D. (1981) The evaluation of short term care for the elderly provided in residential homes, Institute of Biometry and Community Medicine, University of Exeter.
Kushlick, A. and Blunden, R. (1974) Proposals for setting up and evaluation of an experimental service for the elderly, Research Report 107, Health Care Evaluation Team, Winchester.
Kuypers, J. (1972) Internal-external locus of control, ego functioning and personality characteristics in the old, *The Gerontologist*, 12, 168-73.
Lawrence, R. (1982) Domestic space and society: a cross cultural study, *Comparative Studies in Society and History*, 24, 1, 104-30.
Lawson, R. (1992) The mixed economy of residential care, Discussion Paper 841, Personal Social Services Research Unit, University of Kent at Canterbury.
Lawton, M. (1979) Environmental change: the older person as initiator and responder, paper presented at the West Virginia University National Conference on Aging, May.
Lawton, M. (1982) Competence, environmental press and the adaptation of older people, in M. Lawton, P. Windley and T. Byerts (eds) *Aging and the Environment, Theoretical Approaches*, Springer, New York.
Lemke, S. and Moos, R. (1986) Quality of residential settings for elderly adults, *Journal of Gerontology*, 41, 268-76.

Lemke, S. and Moos, R. (1987) Measuring the social climate of congregate residences for older people: Sheltered Care Environment Scale, *Psychology and Aging*, 2, 1, 20-29.

Levin, E. and Moriarty, J. (1990) 'Ready to cope again': breaks for the carers of confused elderly people, National Institute for Social Work Research Unit, London.

Levin, E., Sinclair, I. and Gorbach, P. (1983) *The Supporters of Confused Elderly Persons at Home*, National Institute for Social Work, London.

Levin, E., Sinclair, I. and Gorbach, P. (1989) *Families, Services and Confusion in Old Age*, Gower, Aldershot.

Levin, E., Moriarty, J. and Gorbach, P. (1992) 'I couldn't manage without the breaks': respite services for the carers of confused elderly people, National Institute for Social Work Research Unit, London.

Lewis, J. and Meredith, B. (1989) Contested territory in informal care, in M. Jefferys (ed.) *Growing Old in the Twentieth Century, Routledge*, London.

Lieberman, M. (1961) Relationship of mortality rates to entrance to a home for the aged, *Geriatrics*, 16, 515-19.

Lieberman, M. and Kramer, J. (1991) Factors affecting decisions to institutionalize demented elderly, *The Gerontologist*, 31, 3, 371-4.

Lindesay, J., Briggs, K., Lawes, M., Macdonald, A. and Herzberg, J. (1990) The domus philosophy: a comparative evaluation of a new approach to residential care for the demented elderly, *International Journal of Geriatric Psychiatry*, 6, 727-36.

Lipman, A. (1968) A socio-architectural view of life in three homes for old people, *Gerontologica Clinica*, 10, 88-101.

Lipman, A. (c.1983) Schematic route diagrams, unpublished paper, Welsh School of Architecture, University of Wales Institute of Science and Technology.

Lipman, A. and Harris, H. (1980) Social symbolism and space usage in daily life, *Sociological Review*, 28, 2, 415-28.

Lipman, A. and Slater, R. (1976) Building high to avoid confusing the elderly confused, *Health and Social Service Journal*, 11 September, 1634-5.

Lipman, A. and Slater, R. (1977) Status and spacial appropriation in eight homes for old people, *The Gerontologist*, 17, 250-55.

Lodge, B. (1990) *Alternative Homes for People with Dementia: New Directions in Service Principles and Design*, British Association for Service to the Elderly, Newcastle.

McCormack, D. and Whitehead, A. (1981) The effect of providing recreational activities on the engagement levels of long stay geriatric patients, *Age and Ageing*, 10, 287-91.

Mann, A., Graham, N. and Ashby, D. (1984) Psychiatric illness in residential homes for the elderly: a survey in one London borough, *Age and Aging*, 13, 257-65.

Markson, E. and Cumming, J. (1974) Social consequences of physical impairments in an ageing population, *The Gerontologist*, 9, 39-46.

Marshall, M. (1992) Designing for disorientation, guidelines from the Dementia Services Development Centre, in R. Coles, I. Duncan, M. Kelly, M. Marshall and A. Wightman (eds) *Signposts Not Barriers*, Dementia Services Development Centre, University of Stirling.

Medical Research Council (1987) Report from the MRC Alzheimer's disease workshop, Medical Research Council, London.

Melzer, D. (1990) An evaluation of a respite care unit for elderly people with dementia: framework and some results, *Health Trends*, 2, 64-7.

Millard, P. and Smith, C. (1981) Personal belongings – a positive effect? *The Gerontologist*, 21, 1, 85-90.

Ministry of Health (1955) *Circular 3/55*, HMSO, London.

Ministry of Health (1962) *Local Authority Building Note No 2: Residential Accommodation for Elderly People*, HMSO, London.

Ministry of Health (1973) *Local Authority Building Note No 2: Revision. Residential Accommodation for Elderly People*, HMSO, London.

Moos, R. (1975) Evaluating and changing community settings, *American Journal of Community Psychology*, 4, 313-26.

Moos, R. (1976) *The Human Context: Environmental Determinants of Behaviour*, John Wiley and Sons, Chichester.

Moos, R. and Lemke, S. (1984) *Multiphasic Environmental Assessment Procedure (MEAP) Manual*, Social Ecology Laboratory, Stanford University, Palo Alto, California.

Moos, R. and Lemke, S. (1985) Specialised living environments for older people, in J. Birren and K. Schaie (eds) *Handbook of The Psychology of Aging*, Van Nostrand Reinhold, New York.

Moos, R. and Lemke, S. (1992) *Sheltered Care Environment Scale Manual*, Center for Health Care Evaluation, Department of Veterans Affairs and Stanford University Medical Centers, Palo Alto, California.

Moos, R., Gauvain, M., Lemke, S., Max, W. and Mehren, B. (1979) Assessing the social environments of sheltered care settings, *The Gerontologist*, 19, 74-82.

Morton, J. (ed.)(1991) *Multi-Purpose Homes for Elderly People*, Age Concern, London.

National Health Service and Community Care Act, 1990, HMSO, London.

Neill, J., Sinclair, I., Gorbach, P. and Williams, J. (1988) *A Need for Care? Elderly Applicants for Local Authority Homes*, Avebury/Gower, Aldershot.

Netten, A. (1989) The effect of design of residential homes in creating dependency among confused elderly residents, *International Journal of Geriatric Psychiatry*, 4, 143-53.

Netten, A. (1990) Residential care and senile dementia: the effect of the physical and social environment of homes for elderly people on residents suffering from senile dementia, PhD thesis, University of Kent at Canterbury.

Netten, A. (1991) A positive experience? Assessing the effect of the social environment on demented elderly residents of local authority homes, *Social Work and Social Sciences Review*, 3, 1, 46-62.

Netten, A. (1992) The effect of the social environment on demented elderly people in residential care, in K. Morgan (ed.) *Gerontology: Responding to an Ageing Society*, Jessica Kingsley, London.

Newman, O. (1972) *Defensible Space*, Macmillan, New York.

Newroth, A. and Newroth, S. (1980) *Coping with Alzheimer's Disease: A Growing Concern*, National Institute on Mental Retardation, Downsview, Ontario.

Norman, A. (1984) *Bricks and Mortals: Design and Lifestyle in Old People's Homes*, Centre for Policy on Ageing, London.

Norman, A. (1987) *Severe Dementia: The Provision of Long-Stay Care*, Centre for Policy on Ageing, London.

Nuffield Foundation (1947) *Old People: A Report of a Survey Committee on the Problems of Ageing and the Care of Old People, 1947*, under the chairmanship of B. Seebohm Rowntree. Published 1980 by Nuffield Foundation.

O'Connor, D., Pollitt, P., Hyde, J., Fellows, T., Miller, N., Brook, C., Reiss, B. and Roth, M. (1989) The prevalance of dementia as measured by the Cambridge mental disorders of the elderly examination, *Acta Psychiatr Scand*, 79, 190-98.

Ohta, R. and Ohta, B. (1988) Special units for Alzhiemer's disease patients: a critical look, *The Gerontologist*, 28, 6, 803-8.

Opit, L. (1988) The problems of senile dementia, *Social Behaviour*, 3, 181-96.

Palmore, E. and Luikhert, C. (1972) Health and social factors related to life satisfaction, *Journal of Health and Social Behaviour*, 13, 68-80.

Parker, R. (1981) Tending and social policy, in E. Goldberg and S. Hatch (eds) *A New Look at the Personal Social Services*, Discussion Paper No. 4, Policy Studies Institute, London.

Pastalan, L.A. (1978) Privacy as an expression of human territoriality, in L.A. Pastalan and D.H. Carson (eds) *Spatial Behaviour of Older People*, University of Michigan Press, Ann Arbor, Michigan.

Pastalan, L.A. (1984) Architectural research and life-space changes, in J.C. Snyder (ed.) *Architectural Research*, Van Nostrand Reinhold, New York.

Pattie, A. (1988) Measuring levels of disability: the Clifton Assessment Procedures for the Elderly, in J.P. Wattis and I. Hindmarch (eds) *Psychological Assessment of the Elderly*, Churchill Livingstone, Edinburgh.

Pattie, A. and Gilleard, C. (1975) A brief psychogeriatric assessment schedule: validation against psychiatric diagnosis and discharge from hospital, *British Journal of Psychiatry*, 127, 489-93.

Pattie, A. and Gilleard, C. (1976) The Clifton Assessment Schedule: further validation of a psychogeriatric assessment schedule, *British Journal of Psychiatry*, 129, 68-72.

Pattie, A. and Gilleard, C. (1978) The two year predictive validity of the Clifton Assessment Schedule and the shortened Stockton Geriatric Rating Scale, *British Journal of Psychiatry*, 133, 457-60.

Pattie, A. and Gilliard, C. (1979) *Manual of the Clifton Assessment Procedures for Elderly (CAPE)*, Hodder and Stoughton, London.

Pattie, A. and Moxon, S. (1991) Community units for the elderly in York Health District: an evaluation of the first CUE, Evaluation and Research Support Unit, Psychology Services, Clifton Hospital, York.

Pattie, A., Gilleard, C. and Bell, J. (1979) The relationship of the intellectual and behavioural competence of the elderly and future needs from community, residential and hospital services, research report, Department of Clinical Psychology, Clifton Hospital.

Peace, S. (1986) The design of residential homes: an historical perspective, in K. Judge and I. Sinclair (eds) *Residential Care for Elderly People*, HMSO, London.

Peace, S. and Willcocks, D. (1986) Changing the environment in old people's homes, in K. Judge and I. Sinclair (eds) *Residential Care for Elderly People*, HMSO, London.

Peace, S., Kellaher, L. and Willcocks, D. (1982) A balanced life? A consumer study of residential life in 100 local authority old people's homes, Research Report No. 14, Surrey Research Unit, Polytechnic of North London.

Pollitt, P., Anderson, I. and O'Connor, D. (1991) For better or for worse: the experience of caring for an elderly dementing spouse, *Ageing and Society*, 11, 443-69.

Preston, G. (1986) Dementia in elderly adults: prevalance and institutionalisation, *Journal of Gerontology*, 41, 261-2.

Rabins, P., Merchant, A. and Nestadt, G. (1984) Criteria for diagnosing reversible dementia caused by depression: validation by two-year follow-up, *British Journal of Psychiatry*, 114, 488-92.

Rapoport, A. (1982) *The Meaning of the Built Environment: A Non-Verbal Communication Approach*, Sage, Beverly Hills, California.

Reifler, B., Cox, G. and Hanley, R. (1981) Problems of mentally ill elderly as perceived by patients, families and clinicians, *The Gerontologist*, 21, 165-70.

Residential Care Association (1980) *Staffing Ratios in Residential Homes: A Platform for the 1980s*, Residential Care Association, London.

Retsinas, J. and Garrity, P. (1985) Nursing home friendships, *The Gerontologist*, 25, 418-85.

Robertson, A. (1990) The politics of Alzheimer's disease: a case study in apocalyptic demography, *International Journal of Health Services*, 20, 3, 429-42.

Rodstein, M., Savitsky, E. and Starkaman, R. (1976) Initial adjustment to a long-term care institution: medical and behavioural aspects, *Journal of American Geriatrics Society*, 24, 65-71.

Roth, M. (1955) The natural history of mental disorder in old age, *Journal of Mental Science*, 101, 281-301.

Rothwell, N., Britton, P. and Woods, R. (1983) The effects of group living in a residential home for the elderly, *British Journal of Social Work*, 13, 6, 639-43.

Rovner, B.W., Lucas-Blaustein, J., Folstein, M.F. and Smith, S.W. (1990) Stability over one year in patients admitted to a nursing home dementia unit, *International Journal of Geriatric Psychiatry*, 5, 77-82.

Royal College of Physicians (1981) Organic mental impairment in the elderly, *Journal of the Royal College of Physicians*, 15, 141-67.

Sands, D. and Suzuki, T. (1983) Adult day care for Alzheimer's patients and their families, *The Gerontologist*, 23, 1, 21-3.

Sanford, J. (1975) Tolerance of debility in elderly dependents by supporters at home; its significance for hospital practice, *British Medical Journal*, 3, 471-3.

Schneider, J., Kavanagh, S., Knapp, M.R.J., Beecham, J. and Netten, A. (1992) Elderly people with severe cognitive impairment in England: resource use and costs, Discussion Paper 816, Personal Social Services Research Unit, University of Kent at Canterbury.

Schwab, M., Rader, J. and Dean, J. (1985) Relieving the anxiety and fear in dementia, Journal of Gerontological Nursing, 11, 5, 8-15.

Scottish Action on Dementia (1986) Principles relating to the design of residential environments for dementia sufferers, Discussion Paper, Scottish Action on Dementia, Edinburgh.

Sinclair, I. (1988) Residential care for elderly people, in I. Sinclair (ed.) *Residential Care, The Research Reviewed*, National Institute for Social Work, London.

Snyder, L., Rupprecht, P., Pyrek, J., Brekhus, S. and Moss, T. (1978) Wandering, *The Gerontologist*, 18, 3, 272-80.

Stephens, M. and Willems, E. (1979) Everyday behaviour of older persons in institutional housing: some implications for design, *Environmental Design Research Association*, No. 10, 344-8.

Stephens, M., Kinney, J. and Ogrocki, P. (1991) Stressors and well-being among caregivers in older adults with dementia: the in-home versus nursing home experience, *The Gerontologist*, 31, 2, 217-23.

Stryker, R. (1981) *How to Reduce Employee Turnover in Nursing Homes and Other Health Organisations*, C.C. Thomas, Springfield, Illinois.

Thompson, E.G. and Eastwood, M.R. (1981) Survivorship and senile dementia, *Age and Aging*, 10, 29-32.

Timko, C. and Moos, R. (1991) A typology of social climates in group residential facilities for older people, *Journal of Gerontology*, 46, 3, 160-169.

Tobin, S. and Lieberman, M. (1976) *Last Home for the Aged*, Jossey-Bass, San Francisco, California.

Townsend, P. (1962) *The Last Refuge*, Routledge and Kegan Paul, London.

Townsend, P. (1981) The structured dependency of the elderly, *Ageing and Society*, 1, 1, 5-28.

Wade, B., Finlayson, J., Bell, J., Bowling, A., Bleathman, C., Gilleard, C., Morgan, K., Cole, P., Hammond, M. and Eastman, M. (1986) Drug use in residential settings, in K. Judge and I. Sinclair (eds) *Residential Care for Elderly People*, HMSO, London.

Wagner, G. (1988) *Residential Care: A Positive Choice*, HMSO, London.

West, P., Illsley, R. and Kehman, A. (1984) Public preferences for the care of dependency groups, *Social Science and Medicine*, 18, 4, 287-95.

Wightman, A. (1992) Provision of a caring environment for people with dementia: some design principles: an architect's perspective, in R. Coles, I. Duncan, M. Kelly, M. Marshall and A. Wightman (eds) *Signposts Not Barriers*, Dementia Services Development Centre, University of Stirling.

Wilkin, D. and Hughes, B. (1987) Residential care of elderly people: the consumers' view, *Ageing and Society*, 7, 2, 175-201.

Wilkin, D., Mashiah, R. and Jolley, D. (1978) Changes in behavioural characteristics of elderly population of local authority homes and long stay hospital wards, 1976-7, *British Medical Journal*, 14 November, 1274-6.

Willcocks, D. (1986) Residential homes as community care: a future place for old people's homes in the community they serve, in K. Judge and I. Sinclair (eds) *Residential Care for Elderly People*, HMSO, London.

Willcocks, D., Peace, S., Kellaher, L. with Ring, A. (1982) The residential life of old people: a study of 100 local authority homes, vol. 1, Research Report No 12, Survey Research Unit, Polytechnic of North London.

Willcocks, D., Peace, S. and Kellaher, L. (1987) *Private Lives in Public Places*, Tavistock, London.

Wimo, A., Wallin, J.O., Lundgren, K., Rönnbäck, E., Asplund, K., Mattsson, B. and Krakau, I. (1991) Group living, an alternative for dementia patients: a cost analysis, *International Journal of Geriatric Psychiatry*, 6, 21-9.

Wittels, I. and Botwinick, J. (1974) Survival in relocation, *Journal of Gerontology*, 29, 440-43.

Wolfensberger, W. (1972) *The Principle of Normalization in Human Services*, National Institute on Mental Retardation, Toronto.

Woods, R. (1989) *Alzheimers Disease: Coping with a Living Death*, Souvenir Press, London and Canada.

Woods, R. and Britton, P. (1985) *Clinical Psychology with the Elderly*, Croom Helm, London.

Wyvern Partnership (with University of Birmingham Social Services Unit) (1979) *An Evaluation of the Group Unit Design for Old People's Homes*, Department of Health and Social Security, London.

Subject index

Author Index